C. J. Mathias, P. S. Sever (Eds.)

# Concepts in Hypertension

Festschrift for
Sir Stanley Peart

**Steinkopff Verlag Darmstadt**
**Springer-Verlag New York**

CIP-Titelaufnahme der Deutschen Bibliothek
**Concepts in hypertension** : Festschrift for Sir Stanley Peart / C. J.
Mathias ; P. S. Sever (eds.). – Darmstadt : Steinkopff ; New
York : Springer, 1989
  ISBN 3-7985-0749-X (Steinkopff) Gb.
  ISBN 0-387-91314-9 (Springer) Gb.
NE: Mathias, Christopher [Hrsg.]; Peart, Stanley: Festschrift

Copyright © 1989 by Dr. Dietrich Steinkopff Verlag GmbH & Co. KG, Darmstadt
Medical Editorial: Juliane K. Weller – Copy Editing: Deborah Marston, James Willis – Production: Heinz J. Schäfer

Printed in Germany

Type-setting, printing and bookbinding: Konrad Triltsch GmbH, Würzburg

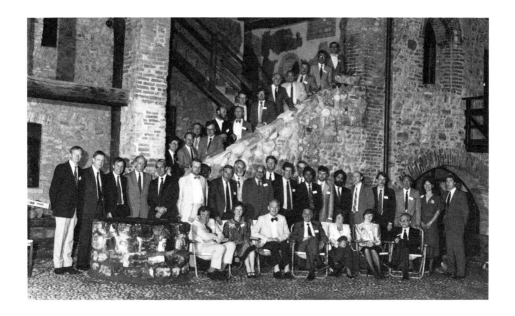

# Foreword

This is a Festschrift to Professor Sir Stanley Peart, Professor of Medicine at St. Mary's Hospital and Medical School, University of London since 1956, who has influenced and directed many of us in the better understanding of the pathophysiological basis and the clinical practice of hypertension. It commemorates, and we hope will preserve, memories of a special occasion when we met to honour him at the Castella de Pomeiro, Como, Italy. At this meeting his "extended family" (pictured above) shared experiences, discussed current scientific and clinical approaches in hypertension research and indulged in reminiscences of their exciting times on his Unit at St. Mary's. We particularly hope that this volume will illustrate the multifaceted approach needed in investigating and managing hypertension and that it will additionally remind Sir Stanley of the admiration and warm affection with which he has been, and will always continue to be regarded.

Christopher J. Mathias
Peter S. Sever

# Introduction

P. S. Sever

Welcome to Castello de Pomerio, for what I feel sure is to be a very special occasion. As all of you know, Stan Peart is retiring after 31 years as professor and head of the department of Medicine at St. Mary's, and after nearly 40 years of distinguished research in basic and clinical science related to the cardiovascular system, the kidney and particularly to hypertension.

His research in hypertension has been exceptional, not only for its quality, which has been outstanding, but also for its breadth and its depth, which have been remarkable. For instance, who could rival a career which began in the late 1940s with the identification of noradrenaline as the sympathetic neuro-effector transmitter; which in the 1950s included the isolation, purification and sequencing of what was then known as hypertension; which has included seminal work on the renin angiotensin and aldosterone system, and which has involved pioneering work in the clinical fields of renal transplantation, renovascular disease and the treatment of mild hypertension?

Chris Mathias and I considered how best we might honour Stan on the occasion of his retirement. Many of you will know by now that we intend to hold a meeting at St. Mary's in his honour. However, we felt that this occasion could not be allowed to pass without a rather different and particularly special meeting – a meeting, which we hope fulfills two main goals: the first is to bring together all of you here today who represent the large number of past and present friends and colleagues who have been associated with Stan on the Medical unit of Mary's, and the second is to hold a meeting which we hope reflects the breadth of his interests in hypertension.

We have had a remarkable response to the invitations that we sent out. Sadly, there were a few who were unable to come, all of whom have expressed their deepest regrets and their hopes that we have a successful day here in Italy. The speakers have all, at one time or another, worked with Stan on the unit, and they span almost the whole period of his time as Professor of Medicine, from Tony Lever at the end of the 1950s through to Mike Taylor, Clive May and Chris Mathias who are present on the unit today. We hope that you will all find the programme both interesting and stimulating.

The choice of chairmen for this afternoons proceedings was not difficult. We could not break a lifetime tradition on the unit of Stan having always the first and the last words. We know that this afternoon he will critically comment upon all the presentations, and I think it is fair to say that he will be ably assisted by Graham Boyd and Alberto Zanchetti.

Finally, some of you will wonder why on earth we are having this meeting in the North of Italy. I suppose by now many of you know of Stan's love for Italy, and particularly, the lakes of the North – what better place therefore to hold this meeting than in Castello de Pomerio, and in association with the third European meeting on hypertension.

# Introduction

C. J. Mathias

As we were drawing up the programme it became abundantly clear to Peter Sever and myself that Stan had influenced hypertension research not only in the United Kingdom and Europe, but all over the world. As we look around here today we most certainly see an international body which I think reflects Stan's ability to attract, to influence and, importantly in my view, to retain the affection of those who have worked with him. This I think is a very special attribute in this outstanding man.

We would not be in this historic and magnificent place if it were not for the very generous support from Boehringer Ingelheim. They have been most kind and helpful and in addition to many in the company, there are two in particular whom I take great pleasure in mentioning – Volker Gladigau and Klaus Schuster, who unfortunately could not be with us today. I am sure you will join me in thanking them for enabling this meeting to proceed in this superb setting. I would also like to thank Alberto Zanchetti and Guiseppe Mancia, who as Chairman and Secretary of the European Society of Hypertension have provided much advice, support and cooperation, and enabled this meeting to be an official satellite of the Milan Hypertension meeting. My warmest thanks to both of them.

Ladies and gentlemen, I am sure that you are all eagerly awaiting the actual start of this meeting and I now hand you over to our Chairman.

# Contents

**Concluding remarks**
Zanchetti, A.   . . . . . . . . . . . . . . . . . . . . . . . . . .   93

**Professional details and bibliography**   . . . . . . . . . . . . . . . . .   97

**After dinner speech**
Grahame-Smith, D. G.   . . . . . . . . . . . . . . . . . . . .   111

**After dinner speech**
Peart, W. S.   . . . . . . . . . . . . . . . . . . . . . . . . . .   117

# Excess renin as a cause of renovascular hypertension?

A. F. Lever

MRC Blood Pressure Unit, Western Infirmary, Glasgow

Ninety years after the discovery of renin we are still not certain whether an excess of the enzyme and its products angiotensins I and II are the cause of renovascular hypertension. Enthusiasm for the idea has been cyclical with research at St. Mary's contributing importantly to the peaks and troughs.

When W. S. Peart became director of the Medical Unit in 1956 the mood was relatively confident. Work by Goldblatt, Pickering, Braun-Menendez, Gross, Wilson and others had established that clipping the renal artery of animals produced sustained hypertension and that the kidneys of animals with renal hypertension contained more renin and released more renin-like enzyme into renal venous blood. It was known that renin was capable of maintaining hypertension on prolonged intravenous infusion in rabbits and Peart (28, 29) had just purified and sequenced angiotensin II which, on a molar basis, was the most potent known vasoconstrictor and pressor agent. All that remained was to show that the concentration of renin and angiotensin II in blood was sufficient to cause the hypertension. No assay at the time had the necessary sensitivity.

Peart, Robertson and Grahame-Smith (30) took a short cut infusing renin into the renal vein of rabbits in a pressor and assayable amount. Measurement of renin in blood downstream showed levels far higher than those in renal venous blood of rabbits with renal hypertension and with similar elevation of blood pressure. Thus, insufficient renin is released into renal venous blood to produce the hypertension via the direct vasoconstrictor effect of angiotensin II.

Perhaps more renin was leaving the kidney in renal lymph (30). Lever and Peart (20) managed to cannulate renal lymphatics and showed that renin and angiotensin did leave the kidney in lymph at a higher concentration than in renal venous blood. They also showed that renal artery constriction increased lymph renin. However, allowing for the tiny volume of lymphatic flow the amount of renin leaving the kidney by this route was still far too small to explain the hypertension. As an interesting side-issue they noted that lymph renin was assayable directly in the rat suggesting a role for renin as an intrarenal hormone.

Meanwhile during the 1960's sensitive methods had been developed at St. Mary's for the measurement of renin (9, 21) and angiotensin II (2) in blood. Work in the Unit with two visiting fellows, Jean-Louis Imbs and Giuseppe Bianchi, showed that the concentration of renin in peripheral blood of hypertensive animals was too small to explain the hypertension by direct vasoconstrictor action of angiotensin II (1, 18, 21). MacDonald, Peart and others (24) reached a similar conclusion when they showed that immunisation of rabbits against angiotensin II did not prevent renal hypertension.

Enthusiasm for the idea of renin as a pressor hormone was now at a low ebb and the decline was hastend by the prospect of an alternative role for renin as a regulator of sodium balance. In the early 1960's, Brown and Peart (11) had established that infusion of angiotensin II in relatively low dose altered urinary sodium excretion. Then, and more or less at the same time in different laboratories, Genest, Laragh, Mulrow and Davis showed that angiotensin II was a stimulant of aldosterone secretion. It remained for Brown and colleagues (7) to show that dietary sodium deprivation stimulated renin and that increased dietary sodium depressed renin. The feedback cycle was now complete: sodium loss probably stimulates renin and angiotensin II which increase aldosterone, causing sodium retention which limits the sodium loss stimulating renin in the first place.

If high sodium suppresses renin, patients with primary hypoaldosteronism (Conn's Syndrome) having expanded body sodium should have abnormally low renin. They did (5, 14), but so did other forms of hypertension without expanded body sodium. Across a wide range of plasma sodium values in hypertensive patients there was an inverse relation with plasma renin concentration (8). At one end were patients with higher renin and lower sodium, some having renovascular disease, at the other end, patients with higher sodium and lower renin, some having mineralocorticoid excess. By 1965 there was more interest in the passive suppression of renin by sodium in hypertension than in the elevation of blood pressure by increased renin. Rightly, the emphasis of research had moved towards the much clearer links of angiotensin with sodium, potassium and corticosteroids (28).

A revival of interest in renin as a pressor agent began just before 1970 when the first renin-secreting tumours were diagnosed (31). The patients had hypertension with increased plasma concentrations of renin and angiotensin II. Removing the tumour reduced renin and angiotensin II and arterial pressure. The tumours contained a very high concentration of renin (10, 31). Nature had provided the best evidence that renin could cause hypertension. Curiously, patients with the tumour had levels of blood pressure and concentrations of renin and angiotensin II which were not markedly different from those in patients with renal artery stenosis (4). In the former renin was considered a cause of the hypertension, in the latter it was thought unimportant.

It had been known for some time that the rise of renin was greatest in the early stages of renal hypertension and that despite the subsequent decrease of renin blood pressure rose progressively thereafter. In 1976 Caravaggi et al. (13) showed that the rise of plasma angiotensin II concentration is sufficient by its direct vasoconstrictor action to explain the early stages of renal hypertension. If excess renin and angiotensin II are the cause of early renal hypertension did they cease to be the cause in the chronic phase? If so, renal hypertension has different causes at different times.

An explanation of the puzzle was suggested by Dickinson and Lawrence (15) who showed that angiotensin II has a second slower-developing pressor action. Prolonged infusion of the peptide at a dose which was at or below the threshold of the direct vasoconstrictor effect produced a gradual but marked rise of blood pressure in rabbits. The response was confirmed in dogs, rats and man. In rats a 50 mm Hg slow pressor effect could be produced by an infusion which had no direct pressor action and which raised plasma angiotensin II concentration 4–6-fold only (3). The mechanism of the slow effect has not been explained. Some evidence suggests that it involves the sympathetic nervous system (16) but other findings are against the idea (25). As angiotensin II has a mitogenic effect on vascular smooth muscle (12, 23) and as vascular hypertrophy is an early feature of renal hypertension the peptide may raise blood pressure by a trophic effect on blood vessels (19). Whatever its mechanism, the importance of the slow effect lies in the ability of a small dose of the peptide to produce a slow-developing but ultimately severe hypertension. Once again angiotensin II had become a candidate for renal hypertension.

Peart has had a longstanding interest in mechanisms controlling release of renin from the juxtaglomerular apparatus of the kidney. By 1974 it was clear that there were three types of stimulus to renin release: a decrease of arterial pressure, sodium loss and increased sympathetic nerve activity. But how are such different stimuli transformed within the JG cell to cause renin release. Peart and Vandongen (29, 32) speculated that *decreased* ionised calcium was the common signal. It was an inspired idea but on the evidence available then it must have seemed mildly eccentric as one by one most other hormones were shown to be stimulated by *increased* intracellular calcium. As it turned out their speculation was correct (17). It explained the origin of the JG cell from vascular smooth muscle, the stimulant effect on renin of vasodilators and beta-adrenergic agonists and the inhibitory effects of increased vascular stretch and of vasoconstrictor agents such as angiotensin II.

W. S. Peart's contributions to the curious cyclical history of research on renin and renal hypertension were to establish the structure and potency of angiotensin II, to be sceptical during a period of false optimism, to encourage work on new and sensitive methods for measuring renin and angiotensin II, to apply these methods in studies of the relation between renin, aldosterone and sodium and to speculate correctly on an unusual and very important cellular mechanism controlling release of renin. We are now on stronger ground in believing that angiotensin II causes renal hypertension, but are still unsure of the mechanism involved.

# References

1. Bianchi G, Brown JJ, Lever AF, Robertson JIS, Roth N (1968) Changes of plasma renin concentration during pressor infusions of renin in the conscious dog.: the influence of dietary sodium intake. Clin Sci 34:303–314
2. Boyd GW, Landon J, Peart WS (1967) Radioimmunoassay for determining plasma levels of angiotensin II in man. Lancet 2:1002–1005
3. Brown AJ, Casals-Stenzel J, Gofford S, Lever AF, Morton JJ (1981) Comparison of fast and slow pressor effects of angiotensin II in the conscious rat. Am J Physiol 241:H381–H388
4. Brown JJ, Bianchi G, Cuesta V, Davies DL, Lever AF, Morton JJ, Padfield PL, Robertson JIS, Schalekamp MAD, Trust P (1976) Mechanism of renal hypertension. Lancet 1:1219–1221
5. Brown JJ, Davies DL, Lever AF, Peart WS, Robertson JIS (1965) Plasma concentration of renin in a patient with Conn's Syndrome with fibrinoid lesions of the renal arterioles: the effect of treatment with spironolactone. J Endocrin 33:279–293
6. Brown JJ, Davies DL, Lever AF, Robertson JIS (1964) Variations in plasma renin concentration in several physiological and pathological states. The Can Med Assoc J 90:201–206
7. Brown JJ, Davies DL, Lever AF, Robertson JIS (1964) Influence of sodium deprivation and loading on the plasma-renin in man. J Physiol 173:408–419
8. Brown JJ, Davies DL, Lever AF, Robertson JIS (1965) Plasma renin concentration in human hypertension: relationship between renin, sodium and potassium. Brit Med J 2:144–148
9. Brown JJ, Davies DL, Lever AF, Robertson JIS, Tree M (1964) The measurement of renin in human plasma. Biochem J 93:594–600

10. Brown JJ, Fraser R, Lever AF, Morton JJ, Robertson JIS, Tree M, Bell PRF, Davidson JK, Ruthven IS (1973) Hypertension and secondary hyperaldsteronism associated with a renin-secreting renal juxtaglomerular-cell tumour. Lancet 2:1228–1232

11. Brown JJ, Peart WS (1962) The effect of angiotensin on urine flow and electrolyte excretion in hypertensive patients. Clin Sci 22:1–17

12. Campbell-Boswell M, Robertson AL (1981) Effects of angiotensin II and vasopressin on human smooth muscle cells *in vitro*. Exper Mol Pathol 35:265–276

13. Caravaggi AM, Bianchi G, Brown JJ, Lever AF, Morton JJ, Powell-Jackson JO, Robertson JIS, Semple PF (1976) Blood pressure and plasma angiotensin II concentration after renal artery constriction and angiotensin infusion in the dog. [5-isoleucine] angiotensin II and its breakdown fragments in dog blood. Circ Res 38:315–321

14. Conn JW, Cohen EL, Rovner DR (1964 b) Suppression of plasma renin activity in primary aldosteronism. J Am Med Ass 190:213–224

15. Dickinson CJ, Lawrence JR (1963) A study developing pressure response to small concentrations of angiotensin. Lancet 1:1354–1356

16. Fink GD, Bruner CA, Mangiapane ML (1987) Area postrema is critical for angiotensin-induced hypotension in rats. Hypertension 9:355–361

17. Fray JCS, Park CS, Valentine AND (1987) Calcium and the control of renin secretion. Endocr Rev 8:53–93

18. Imbs JL, Brown JJ, Davies DL, Lever AF (1967) Plasma renin concentration in conscious rabbits during pressor infusion of renin. Clin Sci 32:83–88

19. Lever AF (1986) Slow pressor mechanisms in hypertension: a role for hypertrophy of resistance vessels? J Hypertension 4:515–524

20. Lever AF, Peart WS (1962) Renin and angiotensin-like activity in renal lymph. J Physiol 160:548–563

21. Lever AF, Robertson JIS (1964) Renin in the plasma of normal and hypertensive rabbits. J Physiol 170:212–218

22. Lever AF, Robertson JIS, Tree M (1964) The estimation of renin in plasma by an enzyme kinetic technique. Biochem J 91:346–352

23. Lyall F, Lever AF, Morton JJ (1988) Vascular hypertrophy of hypertension: a role for growth factors? Acta Physiol Scand 133 (Suppl 571):189–196

24. MacDonald GJ, Louis WJ, Renzini V, Boyd GW, Peart WS (1970) Renal clip hypertension in rabbits immunized against angiotensin II. Circulation Research 27:197–211

25. Ohnishi A, Li P, Branch RA, Holycross B, Jackson EK (1987) Caffeine enhances the slow pressor response to angiotensin II in rats. Evidence for a caffeine-angiotensin II interaction with the sympathetic nervous system. J Clin Invest 80:13–16

26. Peart WS (1955) A new method of large scale preparation of hypertensin with a note on its assay. Biochem J 59:300–302

27. Peart WS (1956) The isolation of hypertensin. Biochem J 62:620–527

28. Peart WS (1965) The renin-angiotensin system. Pharmacol Reviews 17:143–182

29. Peart WS (1977) The kidney as an endocrine organ. Lancet 2:543–548

30. Peart WS, Robertson JIS, Grahame-Smith DG (1961) Examination of relation to renin release of hypertension produced in the rabbit by renal artery constriction. Circulat Res 9:1171–1184

31. Robertson PW, Klidjian A, Harding LK, Walters G, Lee MR, Robb-Smith AHT (1967) Hypertension due to a renin-secreting renal tumour. Am J Med 43:963–976

32. Vandongen R, Peart WS (1974) Calcium dependence of the inhibitory effect of angiotensin on renin secretion in the isolated perfused kidney of the rat. Brit J Pharmacol 50:125–129

Author's address:
Dr. A. F. Lever
MRC Blood Pressure Unit
Western Infirmary
Glasgow G11 6NT
U.K.

# Neuropeptides and renal function:
# The potential for interaction
# between the gastro-intestinal tract and kidney

R. J. Unwin

Dept. of Cellular and Molecular Physiology, Yale University School
of Medicine, New Haven, Connecticut, USA

## Introduction and background

Within the last 10 years, the rapid growth in identification and isolation of "new" gastrointestinal peptides, and the realisation that many, if not all, are in some way related to the central and peripheral nervous systems, have given a new impetus to the field of neuroendocrinology (7, 20, 32); several specialist journals are now devoted almost exclusively to the study of their structure, distribution, pharmacology, and possible physiological functions.

These so-called regulatory neuropeptides, of which some of the better known are listed in Table 1, have been discussed mainly in the context of gastrointestinal function (not unreasonable in view of the origins of many), and nervous system effects. This list is expanding, although many of the newer discoveries are members of established, and structurally related, peptide families, for example, the secretin/glucagon/VIP (vasoactive intestinal polypeptide) and VIP-like group of homologous peptides – see Table 1. The wide distribution of many of these peptides has raised the possibility of physiological roles within other systems, in particular, the respiratory (3, 29) and cardiovascular systems (39), and even the immune system (31): The gastrointestinal tract can safely be described (potentially at least) as the body's most important endocrine organ! Although it is likely that the ubiquity of these peptides reflects nature's tendency to conserve and diversify, the actions and functions, of "useful" chemical substances (c.f. prolactin), and parallel development within tissues, rather than any necessary link between the organs where these substances are

**Table 1.** A list of some established neuropeptides. Those marked with * are also present, or were originally found, in the gastrointestinal tract. Abbreviations are: GRP, gastrin releasing peptide; CCK, cholecystokinin; AVP, arginine vasopressin; NPY, neuropeptide Y (tyrosine, C-terminal amide); PYY, peptide YY; PP, pancreatic polypeptide; VIP, vasoactive intestinal polypeptide; PHI, peptide histidine isoleucine amide; PHM, peptide histidine methionine amide; PHV, prepro-VIP 91-122

| | |
|---|---|
| Angiotensins | *Motilin? |
| Atriopeptins | Neurohypohyseal peptides – AVP/oxytocin/vasotocin |
| *Bombesin/GRP | *Neurokinins – substance P |
| *Endorphins/enkephalins | *Neurotensin |
| *Gastrin/CCK | *NPY, PYY, PP |
| *Insulin? | *Somatostatin |
| Kinins – bradykinin | *VIP, PHI, PHM, PHV, (entero)glucagon, secretin. |

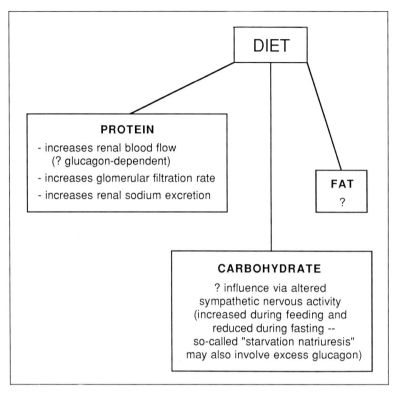

**Fig. 1.** How the main dietary constituents may affect renal function.

found; however, the possibility of such a link should not be ignored, and the concept of an entero-renal interaction, or axis, is certainly worth pursuing. Despite the uncertainty, there may be a more general involvement of the gastrointestinal tract in the regulation of renal function, perhaps more specifically in salt and water homeostasis. After all, in a teleological sense, the gut is daily exposed to a variable amount of dietary sodium and water, and could be the first of many sensors, and regulators, contributing to the control of sodium and water balance (12, 13).

For more than 50 years there has been sporadic interest in various aspects of the relationship between renal function and diet (Fig. 1), from the postprandial rise in renal blood flow and sodium excretion attributed to glucagon, or a glucagon-like, but liver-derived substance (33), and the apparently related adverse effect of dietary protein to increase nephron filtration, ultimately resulting in glomerular injury (as proposed for diabetic glomerulosclerosis) (6); to the postulated enterohepatic or portal osmo-/sodium receptor controlling sodium excretion (25, 26) (though the interest here has been more in terms of sodium loading and natriuresis, rather than sodium depletion and antinatriuresis). Recently, there has been renewed interest in both these aspects of possible gut-kidney interactions, with increased efforts to identify a gut-derived hormone that is able to regulate renal haemodynamics and sodium excretion (33). An added stimulus to this work has come from recent evi-

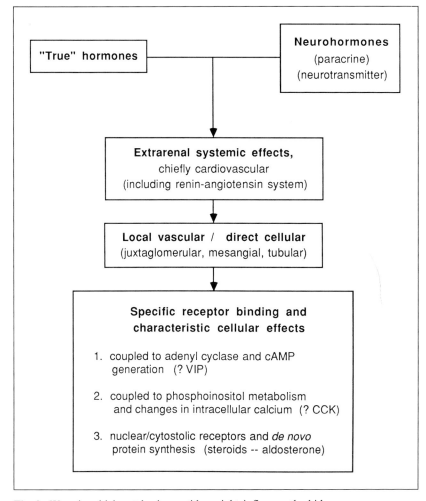

**Fig. 2.** Ways in which gut-brain peptides might influence the kidney.

dence that release of both arginine vasopressin (AVP) and atrial natriuretic peptide (ANP), currently the sodium-regulating neuropeptide *par excellence,* may depend on oropharyngeal stimulation (24): There appears to be an inverse relationship between these hormones.

Neuropeptide hormones may influence renal function at a distance, as true circulating hormones, perhaps released from the gut in response to food and/or its composition, for example, cholecystokinin, gastrin, and neurotensin; or released locally in the kidney as neurotransmitters, with functions quite unrelated to their presence and/or actions within the gastrointestinal tract. Their effects may be extrarenal and indirect, through alterations in systemic haemodynamics, intrarenal, again through vascular changes, or finally, via interactions with specific tissue receptors (Fig. 2) (28).

**Some examples of neuropeptides that affect renal function**

The remainder of this paper is a brief description of some of the diverse renal effects of several gut neuropeptides, as observed in two different species, namely rabbit and man. In fact, the renal actions of 13 "gut-brain" peptides have been studied in the conscious rabbit (gastrin, cholecystokinin, glucagon, vasoactive intestinal polypeptide, neurotensin, pancreatic polypeptide, neuropeptide Y, secretin, substance P, motilin, met-enkephalin, somatostatin and bombesin), but only those which appear to have significant renal effects will be discussed.

Infusion studies, using classical clearance techniques, were performed in conscious rabbits and human volunteers. Experiments in rabbits followed a repeated measurements design (Latin square, or random block), with one control, and 4, or 5, treatments, spanning the physiological-pharmacological dose range; significance was assessed by analysis of variance (4–5 rabbits studied per peptide). Experiments in man comprised a single "off-on-off" infusion protocol; comparisons were made between baseline (control) observations and those obtained during peptide infusion, by paired t-test (six subjects studied per peptide).

*i. Gastrin (as pentagastrin) and cholecystokinin (as the octapeptide, CCK8)*
  (see 10, 20, 32)

I have grouped gastrin and CCK together, because they share the biologically active C-terminal tetrapeptide sequence -trp-met-asp-phe-$NH_2$, and CCK is the established neuropeptide; although CCK8 and gastrin (as the heptadecapeptide, G17) have been identified in both lobes of the pituitary (G17≫CCK8), and could be involved in the regulation of pituitary function.

There appear to be several active forms of CCK: CCK8, ?CCK4 (neural tetrin, about which there is still controversy) and ?CCK12, of which CCK8 is the most abundant form in tissue and plasma. CCK8 is found in proximal gut endocrine cells, and large amounts are present in the central and peripheral (e.g. myenteric plexus) nervous systems, where it can coexist with dopamine, oxytocin, and perhaps even AVP; it has also been found in the urogenital tract, but not the kidney. Thus, there is potential for a dual role as circulating hormone and locally released neurotransmitter.

Figure 3 summarizes the renal actions of intravenously infused gastrin, as pentagastrin, and sulphated CCK8. Pentagastrin exerted a vasopressin-like action in the rabbit, and produced natriuresis in man, with relative sparing of potassium excretion (c.f. the so-called $K^+$-sparing diuretics triamterene and amiloride). Renal haemodynamics did not change, and no changes in plasma AVP concentration were detected. In contrast, in the rabbit, CCK8 decreased plasma calcium concentration (not shown), and was unusual in producing vasodilatation and suppression of plasma renin activity (not shown). In man, its effects were similar to pentagastrin. Both gastrin and cholecystokinin have been implicated in the mesenteric and renal vasodilatation recorded during feeding in dogs, and CCK has been shown to increase circulating levels of calcitonin and parathormone. CCK is known to stimulate pan-

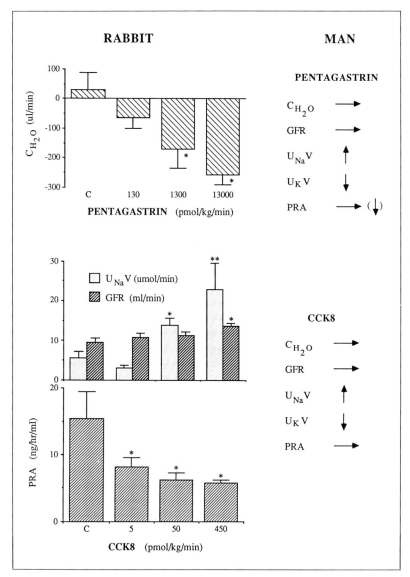

**Fig. 3.** The main renal effects (mean ± S.E.M.) of i.v. pentagastrin and CCK8 in rabbit (left panel) and man (right panel); * and ** indicate $P < 0.05$ and $P < 0.01$, respectively, compared with control, (C). Abbreviations are: ($U_{Na}V$, $U_KV$) renal sodium and potassium excretion, respectively; (GFR) glomerular filtration rate; ($CH_2O$) calculated free water clearance; (PRA) plasma renin activity.

creatic acinar secretion through increased intracellular calcium concentration, and it is conceivable that a similar CCK-related change in cytosolic calcium of renal proximal tubular and juxta-glomerular cells might contribute to the observed natriuresis and renin suppression, respectively (c.f. angiotensin II and proximal tubular function (18)).

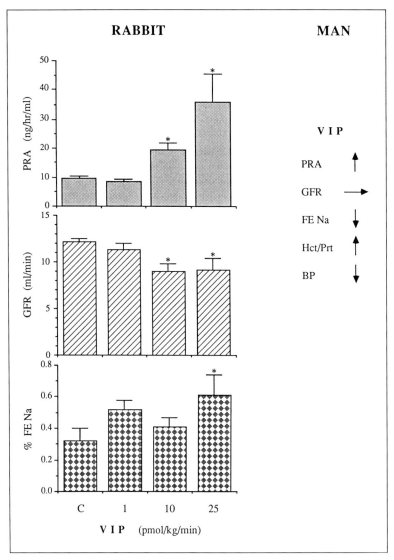

**Fig. 4.** The main renal effects (mean ± S.E.M.) of i.v. VIP in rabbit (left panel) and man (right panel); * indicates P < 0.05 compared with control; (C). Abbreviations are: (FENa) fractional sodium excretion; (GFR) glomerular filtration rate; (PRA) plasma renin activity; (Hct) venous haematocrit; (Prt) plasma proteins; (BP) mean arterial blood pressure.

*ii. Vasoactive intestinal polypeptide (VIP) and related peptides* (see (8, 9, 16, 38))

VIP is found throughout the gastrointestinal tract, and in the central and peripheral nervous systems, particularly in relation to blood vessels. It is believed to be an autonomic neurotransmitter, rather than a circulating hormone, and is a potent vasodilator and smooth muscle relaxant; VIP receptors have also been characterised in cardiac tissue, and linked with increased adenyl cyclase activity (15). Nerve terminals containing VIP-like immunoreactivity have been found in the renal cortex and urogenital tract; in some tissues, for example, salivary glands, VIP can coexist with acetylcholine (4). VIP stimulates sodium and chloride transport in intestinal and renal derived (cultured) epithelium, and the shark rectal gland, where its effect on chloride secretion has been studied in some detail (see (21)).

Figure 4 summarises the renal effects of VIP in rabbit and man. VIP also increased heart rate (not shown) and stimulated renin release, but increased electrolyte excretion (probably through a direct tubular effect – see later) in the rabbit, and reduced it (through a fall in renal perfusion, and haemoconcentration) in man. In the rabbit, the renin response was attenuated by prostaglandin synthetase inhibition with indomethacin, but unaffected by propranolol, suggesting prostaglandin-dependence. In both rabbit and man the tachycardia produced by VIP was blocked by propranolol, indicating beta-adrenoceptor mediation; in man, the cutaneous flush and renin rise were unchanged by either indomethacin or propranolol.

The effects of glucagon in the rabbit were qualitatively similar to those of VIP, except that large doses, as in other species, increased renal blood flow, glomerular filtration rate, and sodium excretion (unpublished observations). Interestingly, as with receptor affinity in rat cardiac tissue (15), the in vitro stimulation of renin release in a crude preparation of glomeruli was, in descending order of potency: secretin, glucagon, VIP (23); perhaps indicating a predominantly "secretinergic" system in rat heart *and* kidney.

### iii. Neurotensin (NT) (see (5, 36))

Originally identified in the hypothalamus, high concentrations have been found throughout the gut, chiefly small bowel, and other regions of the brain. It has a wide variety of central and peripheral nervous system pharmacological effects, including complex dopaminergic interactions (30). There have been reports of NT "receptors" in renal cortical tissue, but not of NT, or NT-like immunoreactivity. Like CCK8, it may also have dual function as hormone and neurotransmitter; but unlike CCK8, there is a very marked postprandial rise (fat is a major stimulus).

When infused in the rabbit NT produced a striking antinatriuresis, apparently independent of changes in glomerular filtration rate and renin release, but only produced a small reduction in chloride excretion in man (Fig. 5). In both species these effects were observed at plasma NT concentrations close to human postprandial levels, but whether, or not, they are functionally significant, is unclear.

### iv. Pancreatic polypeptide (PP) and neuropeptide Y (NPY) (see (1, 2, 17))

Pancreatic polypeptide, as its name implies, is found in the pancreas. Its exact function is uncertain (19); but it is known to stimulate pancreatic exocrine secretion, and may stimulate small bowel electrolyte and water transport (27). However, high circulating levels, as found in some patients with pancreatic endocrine tumours, seem to be without any significant biological effects (19). Blood levels are also high in

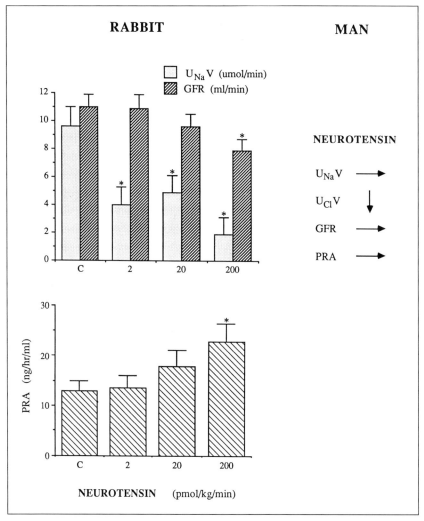

**Fig. 5.** The main renal effects (mean ± S.E.M.) of i.v. neurotensin in rabbit (left panel) and man (right panel); * indicates P < 0.05 compared with control (C). Abbreviations are: ($U_{Na}V$, $U_{Cl}V$) renal sodium and chloride excretion, respectively; (GFR) glomerular filtration rate; (PRA) plasma renin activity.

patients with ileostomies, but this does not appear to be an adaptive response to the increased intestinal losses (37). Because its release is vagally mediated (19), its measurement can be used as an index of vagal activity and an intact vagus, for example, studies of patients with autonomic dysfunction (CJ Mathias, personal communication), or during follow-up of patients who have undergone selective vagotomy for peptic ulceration. In contrast, the closely related peptide NPY is primarily neuronal, and was first isolated from porcine brain and subsequently found throughout the central and peripheral nervous systems (blood vessels, heart and renal cortex) (1, 17). Unlike PP, it is a peripheral adrenergic and noradrenergic co-transmitter, rather

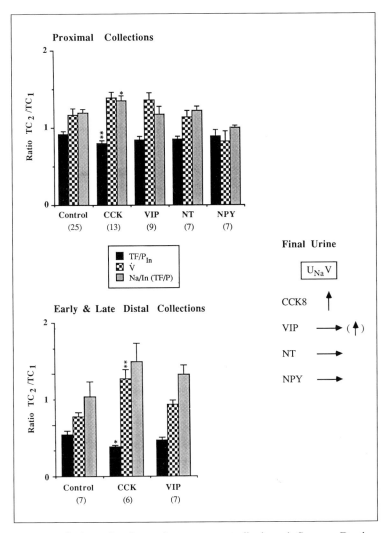

**Fig. 6.** Preliminary data from micropuncture studies in male Sprague-Dawley rats. Results are from recollection experiments; the same tubule sampled twice, the first time during control infusion, and the second time during peptide infusion. Values for tubular fluid insulin concentration/plasma insulin concentration ($TF/P_{In}$), an index of fluid reabsorption, tubular flow rate (V), and fractional delivery of sodium ($Na/In(TF/P)$), are expressed as the ratio of peptide (or control) sample:control sample ($TC_2/TC_1$); number of observations in parentheses. Owing to the small numbers, early and late distal tubule site collections have been grouped together; * and ** indicate $P < 0.05$ and $P < 0.01$, respectively, compared with control ratio. Abbreviations are: (CCK) cholecystokinin octapeptide; (VIP) vasoactive intestinal polypeptide; (NT) neurotensin; (NPY) neuropeptide Y.

than a circulating hormone. It is a potent vasoconstrictor and has been implicated in the pathogenesis of hypertension (1). It has complex, and so far, poorly understood interactions with catecholamines: impaired noradrenaline release, potentiation of noradrenaline-induced vasoconstriction, and a clonidine-like central effect (see (1, 2)).

PP's only renal effect was a fall in renal calcium excretion, which remains an isolated and unexplained finding. In contrast, NPY produced a fall in renal sodium excretion, which was unlike its natriuretic effect in the isolated perfused rat kidney (1), but this was probably due to the associated fall in the glomerular filtration rate – the calculated fractional excretion of sodium did not increase. Mean blood pressure did not rise, but heart rate and plasma renin activity fell; plasma noradrenaline concentrations, an index of sympathetic nervous activity, also appeared to fall slightly, suggesting some inhibition of noradrenaline release. From these differences between the effects of PP and NPY, it might be inferred that the biologically active moiety of the NPY molecule resides more towards its N-terminal end; however one study of N-terminally cleaved NPY fragments in the guinea pig showed significant loss of NPY's cardiovascular effects (35), and the related peptide PYY seems to require an intact amino acid sequence for its vasoconstrictor effect (see (17)). Apart from species variation, the reason for this discrepancy is not apparent.

*v. Possible nephron sites of action for CCK8 and VIP*

Finally, some preliminary results from rat micropuncture studies are illustrated in Fig. 6. These are based on data obtained from recollection experiments (collection from the same accessible cortical nephron segment during i.v. infusion of control and peptide infusates), and indicate some impairment of sodium and water reabsorption in both proximal and distal tubules during CCK8 infusion. Subsequent studies have shown what might be a more localised reduction in sodium and potassium reabsorption within the loop of Henle during systemic infusion of CCK8 *and* VIP (unpublished observations). A more distal site of action for VIP might be important in view of a recent report describing the distribution of VIP-sensitive, and specific, adenyl cyclase along the rabbit nephron (14, 21).

## Conclusion

At this stage is it not possible to state the physiological significance of these findings: apart from NT, changes were observed at supra-physiological plasma concentrations. The fact that they were dose-related, may indicate some relevance to normal function. Some of these peptides could be released locally from renal nerves, and elevated plasma levels have been reported in disease states associated with abnormal renal function, for example, cirrhosis of the liver and VIP (see (11)). Given that the kidney is an important site of excretion and metabolism of several of these peptides, their renal actions may be more important in disease, rather than health (11, 22, 34).

**Acknowledgments**

I would like to thank Professor Sir Stanley Peart, and Dr. David Gordon, for their help and encouragement during the execution of these studies, and Professor G. Giebisch for the opportunity to learn renal micropuncture. I am grateful to Shirley Taylor and Carol Hanson for their excellent technical assistance. The studies in man were carried out in collaboration with Dr. John Calam. My thanks to Amabel Shih for help with the figures. This work was supported by the Medical Research Council and the Wellcome Trust.

## References

1. Allen JM, Bloom SR (1986) Neuropeptide Y: a putative neurotransmitter. Neurochem Int 8:1–8
2. Allen JM, Hanson C, Lee Y, Mattin R, Unwin RJ (1986) Renal effects of the homologous neuropeptides pancreatic polypeptide (PP) and neuropeptide Y (NPY) in conscious rabbits. J Physiol 376:24P
3. Barnes PJ (1987) Regulatory peptides in the respiratory system. Experientia 43:832–839
4. Bartfai T (1985) Presynaptic aspects of the coexistence of classical neurotransmitters and peptides. Trends in Pharmacological Sci 6:331–337
5. Bloom SR, Peart WS, Unwin RJ (1983) Neurotensin and antinatriuresis in the conscious rabbit. Br J Pharm 79:15–18
6. Brenner BM, Meyer TW, Hostetter TH (1982) Dietary protein intake and the progressive nature of kidney disease: The role of hemodynamically mediated glomerular injury in the pathogenesis of progressive glomerulosclerosis in aging, renal ablation, and intrinsic renal disease. New Engl J Med 307:652–659
7. Burgen A, Kosterlitz HW, Iversen LL (eds.) (1980) Neuroactive peptides. Proc R Soc Series B 210:1–195
8. Calam J, Dimaline R, Peart WS, Singh J, Unwin RJ (1983) Effects of vasoactive intestinal polypeptide (VIP) on renal function in man. J Physiol 345:469–475
9. Calam J, Dimaline R, Peart WS, Unwin RJ (1983) Studies on the renin response to vasoactive intestinal polypeptide (VIP) in the conscious rabbit. Br J Pharm 80:13–15
10. Calam J, Gordon D, Peart WS, Taylor SA, Unwin RJ (1987) Renal effects of gastrin C-terminal tetrapeptide (as pentagastrin) and cholecystokinin octapeptide (CCK8) in conscious rabbit and man. Br J Pharm 91:307–314
11. Calam J, Unwin RJ, Singh J, Dorudi S, Peart WS (1984) Renal function during vasoactive intestinal polypeptide (VIP) infusions in normal man and patients with liver disease. Peptides 5:441–443
12. Carey RM (1978) Evidence for a splanchnic sodium input monitor regulating renal sodium excretion in man: Lack of dependence upon aldosterone. Circ Res 43:19–23
13. Carey RM, Smith JR, Ortt EM (1976) Gastrointestinal control of sodium excretion in sodium-depleted conscious rabbits. Am J Physiol 230:1504–1508
14. Charbades D, Griffiths NM, Imbert-Teboul M, Montegut M, Morel F, Simmons NL (1987) Distribution of vasoactive intestinal polypeptide adenylate cyclase activity along the rabbit kidney tubule in vitro. Proc Physiol Soc, September Cambridge Meeting: C37
15. Christophe J, Waelbroeck M, Chatelain P, Robberecht P (1984) Heart receptors for VIP, PHI and secretin are able to active adenylate cyclase ant to mediate inotropic and chronotropic effects. Species variations and physiopathology. Peptides 5:341–353
16. Dimaline R, Peart WS, Unwin RJ (1983) Effects of vasoactive intestinal polypeptide (VIP) on renal function and plasma renin activity in the conscious rabbit. J Physiol 344:379–388
17. Dockray GJ (1986) Neuropeptide Y: In search of a function. Neurochem Int 8:9–11
18. Dominguez JH, Snowdowne KW, Freudenrich CC, Brown T, Borle A (1987) Intracellular messenger for action of angiotensin II on fluid transport in rabbit proximal tubule. Am J Physiol 252:F423–F428
19. Floyd JC (1980) Pancreatic Polypeptide. In: Creutzfeldt W (ed) Clinics in Gastroenterology, Gastrointestinal Hormones. Saunders, London 9:657–678
20. Gregory RA (ed) (1982) Regulatory peptides of gut and brain. Br Med Bull 38:219–318
21. Griffiths NM, Simmons NL (1987) Vasoactive intestinal polypeptide regulation of rabbit renal adenylate cyclase activity in vitro. J Physiol 387:1–17
22. Haffner J, Linnestad P, Schrumpf E, Hanssen LE, Flaten O, Ogasaeter S (1987) The immediate effect of human renal transplantation on basal and meal-stimulated levels of gastrointestinal hormones. Scand J Gastroenterol 22:42–46
23. Hanson C, May CN, Unwin RJ (1987) Effects in vitro of parathormone (PTH) and the homologous peptide family vasoactive intestinal polypeptide (VIP), glucagon and secretin on renin release. J Physiol 382:37P

24. Januszewicz P, Thibault G, Gutowska J, Garcia R, Mercure C, Jolicoeur F, Genest J, Cantin M (1986) Atrial natriuretic factor and vasopressin during dehydration and rehydration in rats. Am J Physiol 251:E497–E501

25. Lennane RJ, Carey RM, Goodwin TJ, Peart WS (1975) A comparison of natriuresis after oral and intravenous sodium loading in sodium depleted man: evidence for a gastrointestinal monitor of sodium intake. Clin Sci Mol Med 49:437–440

26. Lennane RJ, Peart WS, Carey RM, Shaw J (1975) A comparison of natriuresis after oral and intravenous sodium loading in sodium-depleted rabbits: evidence for a gastrointestinal monitor of sodium intake. Clin Sci Mol Med 49:433–436

27. Mitchenere P, Adrian TE, Kirk RM, Bloom SR (1981) Effects of gut regulatory peptides on intestinal luminal fluid in the rat. Life Sci 29:1563–1570

28. Morel F, Doucet A (1986) Hormonal control of the kidney. Physiol Rev 66:377–468

29. Morice A, Sever PS, Unwin RJ (1983) Vasoactive intestinal peptide causes bronchodilatation and protects against histamine-induced bronchoconstriction in asthmatic subjects. Lancet 2:1225–1226

30. Nemeroff CB, Cain ST (1985) Neurotensin-dopamine interactions in the CNS. Trends in Pharmacological Sci 6:201–205

31. O'Dorisio MS, Wood CL, O'Dorisio TM (1985) Vasoactive intestinal polypeptide and neuropeptide modulation of the immune response. J Immunol 135:792s–796s

32. Polak JM (ed) (1987) Regulatory peptides. Experientia 43:723–850

33. Premen AJ (1986) Protein-mediated elevations in renal hemodynamics: existence of a hepatorenal axis? Medical Hypotheses 19:295–309

34. Reed D, Shulkes A, Englin I, Hardy KJ (1986) Neurotensin metabolism in the rat: contribution of the kidney. Aust N Z J Med 16:159

35. Rioux F, Bachelard H, Martel J-C, St.-Pierre S (1986) The vasoconstrictor effect of NPY and related peptides in the guinea pig isolated heart. Peptides 7:27–31

36. Unwin RJ, Calam J, Peart WS, Hanson C, Lee YC, Bloom SR (1987) Renal function during bovine neurotensin infusion in man. Regulatory Peptides 18:29–35

37. Unwin RJ, Moss S, Peart WS, Wadsworth J (1985) Renal adaptation and gut hormone release during sodium restriction in ileostomized man. Clin Sci 69:299–308

38. Unwin RJ, Reed T, Thom S, Peart WS (1987) Effects of indomethacin and DL-propranolol on the cardiovascular and renin responses to vasoactive intestinal polypeptide (VIP) infusion in man. Br J Clin Pharmac 23:523–528

39. Wharton J, Gulbenkian S (1987) Peptides in the mammalian cardiovascular system. Experientia 43:821–832

Author's address:
R. J. Unwin,
Dept. of Cellular and Molecular Physiology,
Yale University School of Medicine,
333 Cedar St.,
New Haven, CT,
USA

# Renin, sodium and hypertension

G. Macdonald

University of New South Wales, School of Medicine,
The Prince Henry Hospital, Little Bay, NSW, Australia

## Introduction

Although the secretion of renin has been shown to be influenced at different levels by many mechanisms – beta adrenergic activity, intracellular calcium concentration, plasma angiotensin II concentration, atrial natriuretic factor, afferent arteriolar distension – regulation of the renin-angiotensin system remains closely linked to sodium metabolism. Its functional activity throughout the body increases in states of sodium depletion and decreases during high dietary sodium intake, administration of mineralocorticoids or other manoeuvres which expand extracellular space.

The direction of changes in blood pressure which accompany such alterations in sodium status are usually opposite to those in renin secretion and the discovery that angiotensin II was the principal stimulus to aldosterone secretion in response to sodium depletion or dietary sodium restriction permitted the elaboration of a theory integrating the three phenomena. Renin was produced by the juxtaglomerular cells of the kidney in response to diminished afferent arteriolar pressure (hypotension, renal artery narrowing, heart failure, apparent intravascular volume contraction in hypo-oncotic states) or to increased sodium concentration at the macula densa. By acting directly or via sympathetic ganglia to constrict arterioles, angiotensin would restore blood pressure (primarily to the kidney and thus to the circulation as a whole). In addition, by acting on the renal tubule or via aldosterone to conserve sodium, it would restore body sodium status, raising blood pressure by extracellular space expansion.

These humoural effects have been held responsible for the development of an ischaemic renal model of high blood pressure and its clinical counterpart, renal artery stenosis. From the outset, it has been difficult to explain why a condition caused by excessive activity of a hormone system is not associated with an increase in circulating hormone concentrations in more than half the patients or experimental animals in which it occurs [2, 17]. The localisation of elements of the renin-angiotensin system and receptors for angiotensin II in the central nervous system and arterial wall [11, 23, 18] and the identification of messenger RNA for renin and angiotensinogen in other tissues [9, 6] has led to the idea of a "whole body" humoral and neurotransmitter system rather than a homeostatic system geared solely to renal perfusion and body sodium conservation. Abnormalities in this expanded system in its various organ sites have been postulated in high blood pressure.

It is difficult to define a set point for an "ideal" total body sodium content in that the sliding inverse relationship between extracellular sodium or volume, blood pressure and plasma concentrations of their principal controlling influence, renin/

angiontensin II/aldosterone remains linear over ranges which extend above and below physiological levels for all three. Insofar as they influence blood pressure, extracellular sodium and volume appear to have the dominant role. Therapeutic reduction in ECF volume (e.g. with diuretic treatment) produces a fall in blood pressure despite a concomitant rise in plasma renin. Effects of sodium depletion external to its effects on renin, perhaps on vascular smooth muscle, reduce the vasoconstrictor effects of angiotensin II.

In some circumstances, both clinical and experimental, this nexus is disrupted. In malignant hypertension in man [3] and the rat, [19] where plasma renin is high, total body sodium is low and further depletion may cause higher blood pressure. Rocchini et al. [20] showed that during the induction of two kidney/one clip renal hypertension in the rat, the renin-stimulating effect of sodium depletion appeared to lead to more severe hypertension than in rats maintained on a normal sodium intake who in turn had higher pressures than rats on a high sodium regime.

It is apparent that more marked degrees of sodium depletion are associated with an inversion of the normal relationship between renin, ECF and blood pressure. The mode of expression of this "resetting" of renin against ECF and blood pressure appears to be by increased renin secretion although other possibilities, such as an increased rate of angiotensin I conversion or altered angiotensin II receptor number or characteristics, have not been explored. Certainly the negative feedback effects of increased circulating angiotensin II on renin secretion seem to be blunted but the responsible mechanism is unknown.

Stan Peart, having been one of the discoverers of angiotensin, was nevertheless a committed sceptic about its role in renal artery clip hypertension. Most of the work I did in his laboratory involved testing this hypothesis, initially, together with Bill Louis and Vincenzo Renzini, in the one kidney-one clip model in the rabbit actively immunised against angiotensin II and then, when the validity of this model was disputed, using passive immunisation in the two kidney-one clip model in the rat. The initiation and maintenance of high blood pressure did not appear to be impaired in any of these studies [16].

The development of peptide analogues of angiotensin II with physiological antagonist properties enabled us to do conventional pharmacological blocking studies in the conscious renal hypertensive rat which showed a strong correlation between induced falls in blood pressure and circulating renin and angiotensin II concentrations [17]. These implied that, at normal concentrations, renin and angiotensin II were not contributing to blood pressure maintenance. Subsequent work indicated that this relationship to prevailing renin or angiotensin II only applies to the acute effects of blockade or converting enzyme inhibition and more chronic administration lowers blood pressure, supposedly "exposing" a dependence on the system [1].

The problem is that this theory demands that angiotensin exert its long-term "conditioning" on the circulation in inverse proportion to its plasma concentration – the acute falls in blood pressure when Saralasin or angiotensin converting enzyme inhibitors are given during high renin states suggest that secondary pressor mechanisms have been induced to a lesser degree than in low renin states, where inhibition or blockade of the system has, by all accounts, little effect.

It can be seen that this problem and the ease with which the elegant control loop for extracellular volume regulation by renin, angiotensin II and aldosterone can be inverted in sodium losing states (or even in a simple rat ischaemic kidney model for hypertension), exposed inadequacies in the original simple but satisfying account of renin, sodium, extracellular space and blood pressure regulation. The first paradox seems satisfied by the re-conception of the renin/angiotensin system in its wider role. The second could not so easily be disposed of.

In the last decade, however, we have for the first time been able to incorporate natriuretic systems into our thinking about blood pressure and volume homeostasis. Atrial natriuretic factor (ANF) was the first of these substances and, like renin and angiotensin, appeared to be a perfectly placed mechanism – intravascular expansion stimulates transformed myocytes in the right atrium to produce ANF, thus correcting the volume change by its natriuretic and vasodepressor properties [12, 10]. The parallel with renin secretion is obvious and many of ANF's actions result from its antagonism to the renin/angiotensin system and its stimulatory mechanisms at every stage [13, 4].

At the moment, to arrive at an integrated hypothesis, it may be necessary to posit some intervening mechanisms in the control of ANF and the renin/angiotensin system or, alternatively, other physiologically significant natriuretic systems. A question which occupied several visiting research workers in the St Mary's laboratory was the question of a monitor for ingested sodium, situated in the upper gut or the portal venous system. It can be shown that, following dietary sodium restriction, natriuresis in the rabbit or man is more rapid after oral repletion with hypertonic saline than after intravenous replacement [14, 15]. If natriuresis depended on the withdrawal of sodium retentive mechanisms brought into play by extracellular contraction, intravascular replacement ought to give more rapid natriuresis. The contrary findings (although not universally agreed to) suggest that there is a natriuretic mechanism *not* dependent on an increase in intravascular volume (i.e. not ANF directly) but released from a site in the upper gut or in the portal vein.

Since early in this decade, workers at St Mary's have shown that many of the active peptides originally identified as "gut hormones" may cause natriuresis when infused in animals [5]. In my own laboratory, Dr Karen Duggan has shown that vasoactive intestinal peptide (VIP) and cholecystokinin octapeptide (CCK8) have this effect when infused directly into the renal artery at doses calculated to deliver physiological concentrations to the kidney while substance P has a species-dependent effect which we believe may depend on the activity of angiotensin converting enzyme [7, 8].

These observations and the discovery of ANF may enable us to explain the apparent discrepancies in the relationship between renin, sodium and hypertension. If the regulation of body sodium is not solely dependent on systems which prevent its excretion, the paradox of volume contracted hypertension may be resolved by the simultaneous activity of a natriuretic system such as ANF in pre-eclamptic toxaemia or malignant hypertension. If, as seems likely, pressor mediators such as angiotensin II and phenylephrine stimulate ANF secretion directly [22], the connection between high blood pressure and natriuresis potentially derives from a much wider base than the intrarenal haemodynamic forces originally postulated by Selkurt [21].

If, in addition, the gastro-intestinal hormones mediate a rapid response monitor for dietary sodium (and we now have evidence that VIP is such a mediator), a more subtle and diverse series of physiological scenarios can be formulated to account for the relationship originally perceived between renin, angiotensin II, aldosterone, body sodium and hypertension as well as the apparent discrepancies. Incorporating an upper gastro-intestinal or portal vein monitor for dietary sodium into theories of sodium metabolism may also bring us closer to an understanding of the part played by dietary sodium in the genesis of essential hypertension. Similarly, recent discoveries about the nature of renin and angiotensin should enable us to account more consistently for their function in the genesis of high blood pressure and disorders of the extracellular space.

## References

1. Bean BL, Brown JJ, Casals-Stenzel J, Fraser R, Lever AF, Morton J, Petch B, Riegger AJC, Robertson JIS, Tree M (1978) An altered relation between arterial pressure and plasma angiotensin II concentration resulting from prolonged infusion of angiotensin II. Clin Sci 55:217S –220S
2. Boyd GW, Adamson AR, Fitz AE, Peart WS (1969) Radioimmunoassay determination of plasma renin activity. Lancet I:213–218
3. Brown JJ, Davies DL, Lever AF, Roberston JIS (1965) Plasma renin concentration in human hypertension. 1. Relationship between renin sodium and potassium. Br Med J 2:144–148
4. Burnett JC, Granger JP, Opgenforth TJ (1984) Effects of synthetic atrial natriuretic factor on renal function and renin release. Am J Physiol 247:F863–F866
5. Calam J, Dimaline R, Peart WS, Singh J, Unwin RJ (1983) Effects of vasoactive intestinal peptide on renal function in man. J Physiol (Lond) 345:469–475
6. Campbell DJ, Bouhnik J, Menard J, Corvol P (1984) Identity of angiotensinogen precursors of rat brain and liver. Nature 308:206–208
7. Duggan KA, Macdonald GJ (1987) Vasoactive intestinal peptide: a direct renal natriuretic substance. Clin Sci 72:195–200
8. Duggan KA, Hams G, Macdonald GJ (1988) Modification of renal and tissue cation transport by cholecystokinin in the rabbit. J Physiol (Lond) 397:527–538
9. Dzau VJ, Ingelfinger J, Pratt RE, Ellison KE (1986) Identification of renin and angiotensinogen messenger RNA sequences in mouse and rat brains. Hypertension 8:544–548
10. Espiner EA, Nicolls GM, Yandle TG, Crozier IG, Cuneo RC, McCormick D, Ikram H (1986) Studies on the secretion, metabolism and action of atrial natriuretic peptide in man. J Hypertens 4 (Suppl 2):S85–S91
11. Ganten D, Schelling P, Vecsei P, Ganten U (1976) Iso-renin of extra-renal origin. Am J Med 60:760–772
12. Gutkowska J, Bourassa M, Roy D, Thibault G, Garcia R, Cantin M, Genest J (1984) Immunoreactive atrial natriuretic factor (IR-ANF) in human plasma. Biochem Biophys Res Commun 123:515–517
13. Harris PJ, Thomas D, Morgan T (1987) Atrial natriuretic peptide angiotensin-stimulated proximal tubular sodium and water sodium reabsorption. Nature 326:697–698
14. Lennane RJ, Peart WS, Carey RM, Shaw J (1975a) A comparison of natriuresis after oral and intravenous sodium loading in sodium-depleted rabbits: evidence for a gastrointestinal or portal monitor of sodium intake. Clin Sci Mol Med 49:433–436
15. Lennane RJ, Carey RM, Goodwin TJ, Peart WS (1975b) A comparison of natriuresis after oral and intravenous sodium loading in sodium-depleted man; evidence for a gastrointestinal or portal monitor of sodium intake. Clin Sci Mol Med 49:437–440
16. Macdonald GJ, Louis WJ, Renzini V, Boyd GW, Peart WS (1970) Renal clip hypertension in the rabbit immunised against angiotensin II. Circ Res 27:197–211
17. Macdonald GJ, Boyd GW, Peart WS (1975) Effect of the angiotensin II blocker 1-sar-8-ala angiotensin II on renal artery clip hypertension in the rat. Circ Res 37:640–646
18. Mendelsohn FAO, Aguilera G, Saavedra JM, Catt KJ (1983) Characteristics and regulation of angiotensin II receptors in pituitary, circumventricular organ and kidney. Clin Exp Hypertens – Theory Prac A5:1081–1097

19. Mohring J, Petri M, Sokol M, Haack D, Mohring B (1976) Effects of saline drinking on malignant course of renal hypertension in rats. Am J Physiol 230:849–857
20. Rocchini AP, Cant JR, Barger AC (1977) Carotid sinus. PA reflexes in dogs with low to high-sodium intake. Am J Physiol 233:H196–H202
21. Selkurt EE (1951) Effect of pulse pressure and mean arterial pressure modification on renal haemodynamics and electrolyte and water excretion. Circulation 4:541–551
22. Shenker Y, Bates ER, Egan BH, Hammoud J, Grekin RJ (1988) Effects of vasopressors on atrial natriuretic factor and haemodynamic function in humans. Hypertension 12:20–25
23. Thurston H, Swales JD, Bing RF, Hurst BL, Marks ES (1979) Vascular renin-like activity and blood pressure maintenance in the rat. Studies of the effect of changes in sodium balance, hypertension and nephrectomy. Hypertension 1:643–649

Author's address:
Graham Macdonald
University of New South Wales
School of Medicine
The Prince Henry Hospital
Little Bay, NSW
Australia

# Inactive renin and the vasculature

G. M. Taylor [1], W. S. Peart [1], H. T. Cook [2]

1 Medical Unit, St. Mary's Hospital Medical School, London, U.K.
2 Department of Experimental Pathology, St. Mary's Hospital Medical School, London, U.K.

## Introduction

Whilst the vasculature is normally considered as a target organ for the circulating renin-angiotensin system, there is growing evidence that the enzyme cascade also exists in blood vessels in man, and that the action of renin on its substrate, angiotensinogen, leads to the local production of angiotensins I and II (ANG-I and ANG-II) within the vessel wall (1, 2, 4). It is proposed that ANG-II produced within resistance vessels could exert local endocrine actions on smooth muscle cells leading to an increase in vascular tone and peripheral resistance. Chronic administration of converting enzyme inhibitors has proved effective in lowering blood pressure in a high proportion of patients with essential hypertension and in certain animal models of hypertension where plasma renin activity may be near normal. This has led to speculation as to the involvement of the vascular renin-angiotensin system in essential hypertension, in the spontaneously hypertensive rat strain and in the 2-kidney 1-clip animal model of renal artery stenosis (4). There is also evidence to suggest that ANG-II acts via pre-junctional receptors at local sympathetic nerve endings to facilitate sympathetic neurotransmission (15, 16).

Fernandez and colleagues have shown that administration of ANG-II into the rabbit cornea results in the formation of new blood vessels (8), suggesting angiotensin II may also be one of the growth factors involved in the process of neovascularization. There is also interest in the renin-angiotensin system as a mediator of the formation of collateral vessels which occurs in ischaemic kidneys (9, 14). Thus, more widespread roles for the extrarenal vascular renin-angiotensin system may include involvement in other conditions where there is new vessel formation, such as wound healing and the inflammatory response: earlier in vitro experiments have shown that activation of the factors of the intrinsic haemostatic pathway, which occurs in the inflammatory response, may result in the activation of inactive plasma renin (18), a circulating precursor of renin which has many biochemical similarities with kidney renin. One role for the system may therefore be as part of the local response to tissue injury to restrict haemorrhage through the vasoconstrictor actions of ANG-II at times when the clotting system is activated.

In addition to the local endocrine actions of renin and angiotensin, it is proposed that all the components of the system may be present in many cell types and that ANG-II may be produced, and act, intracellularly. Intracellular ANG-II acceptor sites have been described on mitochondria and nuclear chromatin (20). Putative actions of ANG-II produced within cells include specific gene activation and regulation of protein synthesis (19). In addition, Ang-II has been reported to be a mitogen for some cell types in culture, such as mouse 3T3 cells (11) and the data presented by Lever in this volume suggests that this may also be true for rat vascular smooth muscle cells.

## Vascular renin in man

The presence of renin has been reported in a large number of normal extrarenal tissues and in certain pathological conditions, often associated with vessels or vascular spaces (Table 1). There is both immunohistochemical and biochemical evidence for the presence of renin in arteries (5). However, extracts of arterial tissues also contain other proteases, probably of lysosomal origin like cathepsin D, which may also generate ANG-I, or tonin capable of forming ANG-II directly from renin substrate (12). Therefore, any study seeking to demonstrate renin in these tissues must distinguish the non-specific renin-like activity from renin itself. It is not clear whether the renin which exists in blood vessels in man is present as a result of local synthesis or uptake from the plasma or a combination of these processes. There is evidence to suggest that at least part of the vascular renin in some animal species is present as a result of uptake (22).

It is often quoted that, in man, up to 90% of renin in plasma may be in the inactive, HMW form (21). In theory this represents a circulating pool from which renin could undergo selective uptake into vessels and conversion to an enzymatically active form by proteases within vascular endothelial cells, and models for this process have been proposed (6).

The local production within the vessel wall of ANG-II would require the presence of angiotensinogen, the substrate of renin, a glycoprotein of approximately 64,000 daltons molecular size. Like renin, angiotensinogen in the vessel wall may be the result of uptake or synthesis, or a combination of both processes. Little is known of local angiotensinogen production in man, but the possibility of extrahepatic synthesis has been demonstrated in various tissues in the rat and mouse, including the aorta, using cDNA probes for angiotensinogen mRNA (7, 17).

Two rare but interesting pathological conditions have been linked with inappropriate extrarenal renin production (Table 1). These are worthy of mention due to their association with blood vessels. They are: (1) Alveolar soft part sarcoma (ASPS) a malignant angioreninoma involving soft tissues. Whilst the exact classification of this neoplasm has remained a matter of dispute, the cells comprising the tumour are

**Table 1.** Extrarenal renin in man

| | |
|---|---|
| 1. In tissue extracts ............... | Adrenal, brain, uterus, ovary, placenta, amniotic fluid, blood vessel wall. |
| 2. Cells in culture ................. | Neuroblastoma × glioma cells, mesangial cells, juxtaglomerular cells, smooth muscle cells. |
| 3. Immunoreactive renin ........... | Ant. pituitary, testis, thyroid, prostate, blood vessels. |
| 4. Pathological conditions .......... | Renin-secreting tumours, alveolar soft-part sarcoma (ASPS), angiolymphoid hyperplasia with eosinophilia (ALHE). |

believed to be modified smooth muscle cells, and, like the juxtaglomerular cells in the kidney, cells lining vascular spaces in these tumours contain characteristic secretory storage granules which stain positively for renin (3). Primary reninism with hypertension has not been reported in ASPS, which implies that either renin does not reach the circulation or that a biologically inactive form is produced.

The second condition is angiolymphoid hyperplasia with eosinophilia (ALHE, Table 1), a reactive inflammatory condition of unknown cause involving the skin and subcutaneous tissues. The lesions in ALHE are usually at sites in the neck or head and are characterised by marked vascular proliferation. A syndrome of primary reninism has been reported in ALHE (10). This resolved upon surgical removal of the mass. The presence of immunoreactive vascular renin was noted by the authors in a total of 6 out of 8 further cases studied, but was not associated with increased plasma renin activity (10).

## Properties of vascular renin

### (a) Human fetal lung

At the Medical Unit at St. Mary's, we have been interested in two further conditions in which we find that new vessel formation, as in ALHE, is associated with the presence of renin in the vessel wall. We have observed that extracts of human fetal lung between gestational ages of approximately 10–20 weeks contain an inactive form of renin which may be revealed by trypsin treatment of crude homogenates. This is shown in Fig. 1. Untrypsinized fetal lung homogenates contained undetectable or low basal levels of renin-like activity. Figure 1 also shows the effect of a specific MC antibody, R-3-36-16, raised to human kidney renin which abolished the increase in renin activity seen after trypsin treatment but had no effect on the "renin-like" activity, suggesting this was due to other proteases in the lung.

Using a sensitive alkaline phosphatase-anti-alkaline phosphatase (APAAP) immunohistochemical procedure for renin (23), the form in fetal lung has been localized in the cytoplasm of single cells or in cords of cells in the mesenchyme surrounding the developing fetal airways (Fig. 2). The staining was often present in a branching pattern and in some cases was clearly in the cytoplasm of cells in the walls of blood vessels. This pattern of staining was found in nine out of 14 cases studied. A very similar pattern was seen when the same blocks of tissue were examined for Factor VIII-related antigen, a marker for endothelial cells, and it seems likely that the appearances of renin staining in the fetal lung are consistent with its localization in the vascular endothelial cells.

### (b) Human pulmonary tumours

We have also found that renin may be readily demonstrated in blood vessels in human pulmonary tumours using the same localization procedure on formalin-fixed and routinely-processed tissue. Table 2 shows the incidence of immunoreactive renin in the various categories of tumours examined. The most strongly positive staining

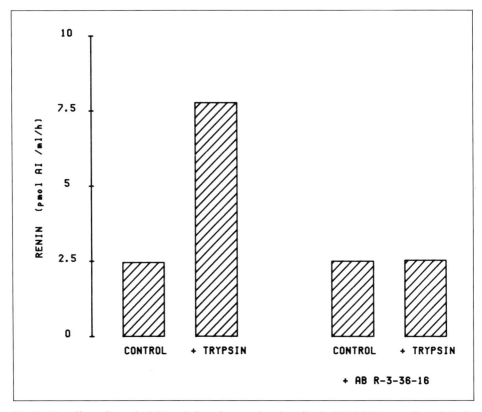

**Fig. 1.** The effect of trypsin (400 µg/ml) and monoclonal antibody R-3-36-16 on renin activity in human fetal lung homogenate.

**Table 2.** Categories of human pulmonary tumours studied and the incidence of immunoreactive renin in tumour vessel walls

| Tumour category | Cases studied | Immunoreactive renin |
|---|---|---|
| Adenocarcinoma | 18 | 15 |
| Squamous cell | 8 | 7 |
| Undifferentiated large cell | 4 | 4 |
| Undifferentiated small cell | 1 | 1 |
| Carcinoid | 1 | 1 |
| Atypical small cell | 1 | 0 |
| Bronchioloalveolar cell tumour (BACT) | 3 | 0 |
| Total | 36 | 28 (78%) |

was seen in adenocarcinomas. Squamous cell carcinomas were frequently positive but the intensity of staining rarely matched that of the former category. Within the tumours, renin was present in the walls of arterioles ranging in size from approximately 50–250 µM. The most intense staining was often noted in the inflamed regions of fibrous tissue at the borders of the tumour and lung, rather than in the

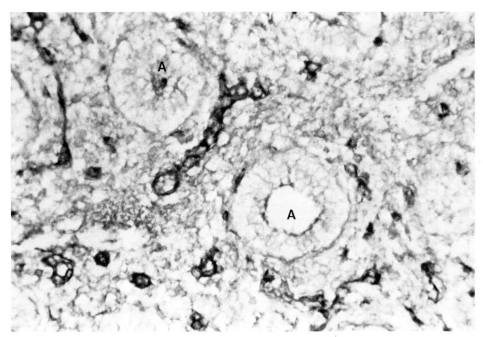

**Fig. 2.** Immunoreactive renin localized by the APAAP method (see text) in the developing vasculature surrounding primitive airways (A) in human fetal lung of gestational age 15 weeks. Magnification × 450, Haematoxylin counterstain.

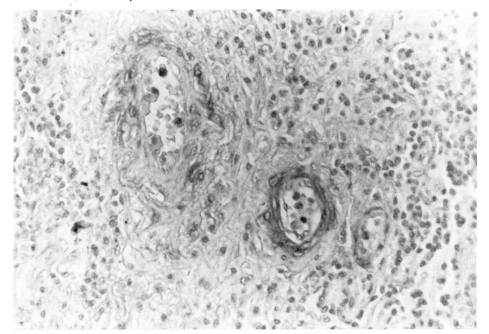

**Fig. 3.** Vascular renin staining in human pulmonary adenocarcinoma. Staining is present in a group of vessels in an inflamed region at the boundary of the tumour and lung. Magnification × 350. Haematoxylin counterstain.

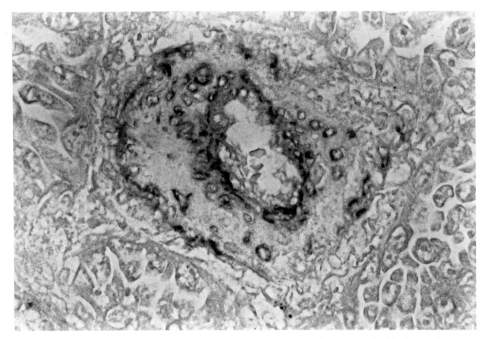

**Fig. 4.** Vascular renin staining in human pulmonary adenocarcinoma. A double layer of renin-positive cells are seen in the wall of an arteriole within the tumour. Magnification × 705, Haematoxylin counterstain.

body of the tumour itself (Fig. 3). In these inflamed regions, staining was often in groups of vessels. In the vessels themselves, renin was localized in the cytoplasm of smooth muscle cells in the media of the arterioles. In several cases, staining was observed in a double layer of cells, one immediately below the endothelium and the other at the outer edge of the media, which had a thickened appearance (Fig. 4). Not all arterioles within the tumour itself or in the inflamed regions stained positively, suggesting synthesis or uptake of renin was occurring in selected vessels only.

Staining for vascular renin in both fetal lung and lung tumour sections was either significantly reduced or abolished when the primary antibody R-15 was preincubated with purified human kidney renin before use and was absent when "irrelevant" primary rabbit anti-human antisera were substituted for the renin antibody.

Immunoaffinity chromatography using MC antibodies R-3-36-16 and R-3-27-6 (13) coupled to Sepharose have been used to extract renin from lung tumour extracts, prepared from tissue obtained at operation from patients undergoing surgical resection of the lung for adenocarcinoma, or from fetal abortuses. Low levels of renin with biological activity and an inactive form of renin were present in tumour extracts. Gel filtration of immunoaffinity purified renins on Sephadex G 100 Superfine showed that the MW of both active and inactive renin in the tumours and of inactive renin in fetal lung was HMW, approximately 56,000 daltons. In contrast, the MW of inactive renin purified from fetal kidney was 45,000 daltons, significantly less than the vascular renin. The reasons for this difference in MW remain unresolved. Activation of vascular inactive renin was not accompanied by any discernible reduction in

MW. We know from previous studies that activation of fetal kidney inactive renin does not result in any detectable shift in MW (24). This would imply that the MW of the sequence cleaved from the precursor molecules in both cases is within the limits of detection of the column (10%). Preliminary studies have shown that the inactive HMW vascular renin has biochemical similarities to plasma inactive renin in man. Both are of similar MW, are bound to Affigel Blue affinity chromatography resin, may be activated by exogenous trypsin with little or no reduction in MW, have a pH optimum of approximately 6.5 and are bound and inhibited by MC antibodies (R-3-36-16 and R-3-27-6) raised to human kidney renin. Many of these biochemical characteristics are shared by the inactive form of renin which we have studied in the plasma of long-term anephric patients (25), which would support the suggestion made by various workers that the vasculature is one possible source of circulating HMW inactive renin in man.

# References

1. Caldwell PRB, Seegal BC, Hsu KC (1976) Angiotensin converting enzyme: vascular endothelial localization. Science 191:1050–1051
2. Campbell DJ (1985) The site of angiotensin production. J Hypertens 3:199–207
3. De Schryver-Kecksmeti K, Kraus FT, Engleman W, Lacey PE (1982). Alveolar soft-part sarcoma – A malignant angioreninoma. Am J Surg Pathol 6:5–18
4. Dzau VJ (1984) Vascular wall renin-angiotensin pathway in control of the circulation: a hypothesis. Am J Med 77 (Suppl 4A):31–36
5. Dzau VJ (1987) Implications of local angiotensin production in cardiovascular physiology and pharmacology. Am J Cardiol 59:59A–65A
6. Dzau VJ (1987) Possible prorenin activating mechanisms in the blood vessel wall. J Hypertens 5 (Suppl 2):S15–S18
7. Eggena P, Barrett JD, Fredal AM, Morin AM (1987) Stimulation of brain and aortic renin substrate by central administration of steroids in the rat. J Hypertens 5 (Suppl 2):S11–S13
8. Fernandez LA, Twickler J, Mead A (1985) Neovascularization produced by angiotensin II. J Lab Clin Med 105:141–145.
9. Fernandez LA, Caride VJ, Twickler J, Galardy RE (1982) Renin-angiotensin and development of collateral circulation after renal ischaemia. Am J Physiol 243 (Heart Circ Physiol 12):H869–H875
10. Fernandez LA, Olsen TG, Barwick KW, Sanders M, Kaliszewski C, Inagami T (1986) Renin in angiolymphoid hyperplasia with eosinophilia. Arch Pathol Lab Med 110:1131–1135
11. Ganten D, Schelling P, Flugel RM, Fischer H (1975) Effect of angiotensin and the angiotensin antagonist P113 on iso-renin and cell growth in 3T3 mouse cells. Int. Res. Commun. Med. Sci. 3:327
12. Genest J, Garcia R, Thibault G et al. (1981) The present status of the tonin-angiotensin II system. In: Sambhi MP (ed) Heterogeneity of Renin and Renin-Substrate. Elsevier, North-Holland, pp 11–24
13. Heusser ChH, Bewes JPA, Alkan SS, Dietrich FM, Wood JM, de Gasparro M, Hofbauer KG (1987) Monoclonal antibodies to human renin. Properties and applications. Clin Exper-Theory Pract A9 (8 and 9):1259–1275
14. Hollenberg NK, Paskins-Hurlburt AJ, Abrahams HL (1985) Collateral arterial formation: Lymph draining ischaemic kidneys contains a neovascular stimulating agent of high molecular weight. Invest Radiol 20:58–61
15. Kawasaki H, Cline WH, Che Su (1984) Involvement of the vascular renin-angiotensin system in Beta adrenergic receptor-mediated facilitation of vascular neurotransmission in spontaneously hypertensive rats. J Pharmac Exp Ther 231:23–32
16. Nakamaru M, Jackson EK, Inagami T (1986) Beta adrenoreceptor-mediated release of angiotensin II from mesenteric arteries. Am J Physiol 250 (Heart Circ Physiol 19):H144–H148

17. Ohkubo H, Nakayama K, Tanaka T, Nakanishi S (1986) Tissue distribution of rat angiotensinogen mRNA and structural analysis of its heterogeneity. J Biol Chem 261:319–323
18. Osmond DH, Tatemichi SR, Wilczynski EA, Purdon AD (1981) Coagulation and fibrinolytic enzymes as co-activators of human plasma renin. In: Sambhi MP (ed) Heterogeneity of Renin and Renin-Substrate. Elsevier, North-Holland, pp 139–157
19. Re R, Parab M (1983) Effect of angiotensin II on RNA synthesis by isolated nuclei. Life Sciences 34:647–651
20. Robertson AL, Khairallah PA (1971) Angiotensin: Rapid localization in nuclei of smooth and cardiac muscle. Science 172:1138–1140
21. Sealey JE, Atlas SA, Laragh JH (1980). Prorenin and other large molecular weight forms of renin. Endocr Rev 1:365–391
22. Swales JD; Abramovici A, Beck F, Bing RF, Loudon M, Thurston H (1983) Arterial wall renin. J Hypertens 1 (Suppl 1):17–22
23. Taylor GM, Cook HT, Sheffield EA, Hanson C, Peart WS (1988) Renin in human pulmonary tumours: An immunohistochemical and biochemical study. Am J Pathol 130:543
24. Taylor GM, Peart WS, Porter KA, Zondek LH, Zondek T (1986) Concentration and molecular forms of active and inactive renin in human fetal kidney, amniotic fluid and adrenal gland: Evidence for renin-angiotensin system hyperactivity in 2nd trimester of pregnancy. J Hypertens 4:121–129
25. Taylor GM, Carmichael DJS, Peart WS (1986) Active and inactive renin in anephric man: A comparison of molecular weight studies with normal human plasma and the effect of a specific monoclonal anti renin antibody. J Hypertens 4:703–712

Authors' address:
Dr. G. M. Taylor,
Medical Unit,
St. Mary's Hospital Medical School,
Norfolk Place,
London W2 1PG,
U.K.

# Investigation of the mechanisms by which angiotensin II and isoprenaline alter calcium flux in juxtaglomerular cells

C. N. May and Sir Stanley Peart

Medical Unit, St. Mary's Hospital Medical School, London, U.K.

## Introduction

A central role for $Ca^{2+}$ in stimulus-secretion coupling has been demonstrated in many secretory systems. Generally, an increase in intracellular $Ca^{2+}$ stimulates secretion, but studies by Peart and colleagues suggested that the opposite may be true for renin. It was known that in smooth muscle cells, from which juxtaglomerular cells are thought to be derived (1), an increase in intracellular $Ca^{2+}$ produced contraction (2). The possibility that changes in $Ca^{2+}$ flux in JG cells may alter renin secretion was investigated in a series of studies using the isolated perfused kidney.

Angiotensin II (AII) inhibited basal and isoprenaline stimulated renin secretion from the isolated kidney when $Ca^{2+}$ was present in the perfusion fluid (Fig. 1) (17). In the absence of $Ca^{2+}$ the inhibitory effect of AII was abolished, suggesting that it acts by increasing $Ca^{2+}$ flux into cells. The effect of increasing intracellular $Ca^{2+}$ was demonstrated using the $Ca^{2+}$ ionophore A23187, which produced a fall in renin secretion together with vasoconstriction (8). These changes were dependent on extracellular $Ca^{2+}$, demonstrating that they resulted from influx of $Ca^{2+}$ into the cells. Conversely, reducing intracellular $Ca^{2+}$ by chelation of $Ca^{2+}$ in the perfusate with

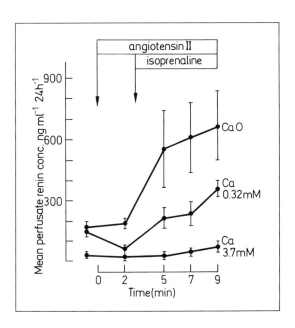

Fig. 1. The effect of AII on basal and isoprenaline stimulated renin release in the presence of $Ca^{2+}$ (3.7 mM and 0.32 mM) and in the absence of $Ca^{2+}$. Angiotensin (6 mg/min/g) was started at 0 min and isoprenaline (0.01 µg/min/g) at 3 min.

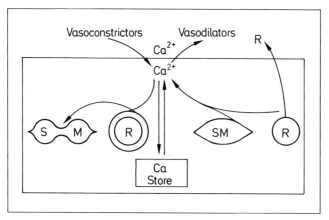

**Fig. 2.** Diagrammatic representation of calcium flux hypothesis relating renin release (R) and arteriolar smooth-muscle contraction (SM).

(Left): Influx of calcium leading to increased intracellular ionised calcium ($Ca^{2+}$) causes, on the one hand, smooth-muscle contraction, and on the other, inhibition of renin release. (Right): Efflux of calcium leading to reduction of intracellular ionised calcium causes smooth-muscle relaxation and increased release of renin.

EDTA produced increases in renin secretion and vasodilatation (16). These findings were the basis of the calcium flux hypothesis which suggested that a decrease in intracellular $Ca^{2+}$ led to stimulation of renin secretion and vasodilatation, while the opposite, an increase in intracellular $Ca^{2+}$ caused inhibition of renin secretion and vasoconstriction (Fig. 2) (15).

In these studies, agents which altered renin secretion also produced haemodynamic changes which may have affected secretion. To avoid this an in vitro rat kidney cortex preparation was developed and the mechanisms by which AII inhibits, and β-adrenergic agonists stimulate, renin secretion were investigated.

### Renal cortex preparation

This was prepared as previously described (12). Briefly, cortex from two rat kidneys was broken up on a 350 μm sieve, divided into twelve equal lots and placed in 4 ml plastic tubes. These contained 2 ml of incubation medium; (mM) NaCl 118.5, $NaHCO_3$ 24.9, KCl 5.9, $CaCl_2$ 2.54, $NaH_2PO_4$ 1.18, glucose 10 and bovine serum albumin 0.5%. The tubes were flushed with 95% $O_2$ 5% $CO_2$ and capped. The tissue was incubated at 37 °C and at the end of each 15-min incubation period the tubes were gently shaken, centrifuged at 100 g for 1 min and fresh incubation medium added. The supernatant from the first four incubation periods was discarded. From subsequent supernatants a sample was taken for the measurement of renin activity (12).

Renin secretion is expressed as the percentage change from the baseline level measured in the first incubation period. The results are presented as the mean ±SEM of six observations. Unpaired Student's $t$-test was used to assess the statistical significance of differences due to treatment.

### Effect of AII and ouabain on renin secretion

Using this preparation basal renin release from renal cortex incubated in normal medium (2.5 mM $Ca^{2+}$) fell with time, and addition of AII ($10^{-5}$ M) or ouabain ($5 \times 10^{-4}$ M) inhibited renin secretion (Fig. 3a). In the absence of $Ca^{2+}$ in the medium the inhibitory effects of both AII and ouabain were abolished (Fig. 3b), indicating that they cause $Ca^{2+}$ flux into JG cells which raises intracellular $Ca^{2+}$ and inhibits renin secretion. This confirms the findings in the isolated kidney and demonstrates that the inhibition of renin secretion is due to a direct effect of AII on JG cells and is not a result of haemodynamic changes.

### *β-adrenergic stimulation of renin release*

It is thought that $β$-adrenoceptor agonists stimulate renin secretion by reducing intracellular $Ca^{2+}$ since manoeuvers which cause $Ca^{2+}$ influx antagonise the effects of isoprenaline (3). The effects of $β$-adrenoceptor agonists are mediated by an increase in cAMP but how this leads to alterations in $Ca^{2+}$ flux and renin secretion is unclear.

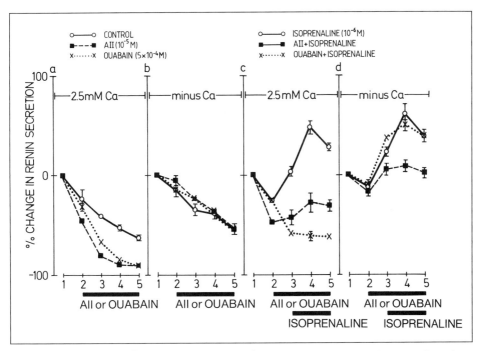

**Fig. 3.** Effect of AII ($10^{-5}$ M) or ouabain ($5 \times 10^{-4}$ M) on basal (a and b) and isoprenaline stimulated (c and d) renin secretion from rat kidney cortex incubated in normal 2.5 mM medium (a and c) or in $Ca^{2+}$ free medium (b and d). Means are shown with SEM indicated by a vertical line, except where it is less than the symbol size. (Reproduced with permission from the British Journal of Pharmacology, as in ref. (12)).

Isoprenaline ($10^{-6}$ M) significantly increased renin secretion from tissue incubated in normal medium (Fig. 3c). Addition of AII for one incubation period before and then together with isoprenaline significantly reduced the increase in renin secretion from tissue incubated in normal medium (Fig. 3c). Likewise, ouabain significantly reduced the stimulation of renin secretion by isoprenaline in normal medium (Fig. 3c). These findings confirm those of Churchill and Churchill (3), that agents which increase intracellular $Ca^{2+}$ inhibit isoprenaline stimulated renin secretion, indicating that isoprenaline acts by reducing intracellular $Ca^{2+}$.

Addition of isoprenaline to renal cortex incubated in $Ca^{2+}$ free medium resulted in a similar increase in renin secretion to that seen in normal medium (Fig. 3d). In $Ca^{2+}$ free medium AII inhibition of isoprenaline stimulated renin secretion was attenuated but not abolished, in contrast to its inhibitory effect on basal renin release which was absolished in the absence of $Ca^{2+}$. The ability of AII to reduce isoprenaline stimulated renin secretion in the absence of extracellular $Ca^{2+}$ suggests that two mechanisms are involved; one dependent on extracellular $Ca^{2+}$ and the other independent. The component dependent on extracellular $Ca^{2+}$ probably results from stimulation of $Ca^{2+}$ influx as has been shown for AII in smooth muscle cells (2). The reduction of isoprenaline stimulated renin secretion in $Ca^{2+}$ free medium could depend on the release of $Ca^{2+}$ from intracellular storage sites. An alternative or additional mechanism is that AII may attenuate the action of isoprenaline by inhibition of adenyl cyclase as has been reported in membranes from other tissues including kidney (18) and pituitary (13). Further evidence that AII acts on adenyl cyclase is the demonstration that pretreatment with pertussis toxin, which inactivates the inhibitory protein ($N_1$) that mediates receptor-induced inhibition of adenyl cyclase, attenuates the inhibition of renin secretion by AII (9).

The inhibitory effect of ouabain ($5 \times 10^{-4}$ M) on isoprenaline stimulated renin release was abolished in the absence of $Ca^{2+}$ (Fig. 3d). Thus, in the absence of extracellular $Ca^{2+}$, isoprenaline stimulates renin secretion when the $Na^+/K^+$-ATPase is blocked with ouabain. This does not support the suggestion that $\beta$-agonists increase renin secretion by stimulating $Na^+/K^+$-ATPase and indirectly causing $Ca^{2+}$ efflux via $Na^+ - Ca^{2+}$ exchange (4, 6). In JG cells, isoprenaline must increase $Ca^{2+}$ efflux via a different mechanism and may also cause uptake of $Ca^{2+}$ into intracellular stores.

## $Ca^{2+}$ flux across potential dependent channels in JG cells

Basal renin secretion was increased by verapamil ($5 \times 10^{-6}$ M) in normal medium but not in the absence of $Ca^{2+}$ (Fig. 4a, b), suggesting that there is a basal influx of $Ca^{2+}$ through potential dependent channels. The inhibition of renin secretion by AII was not prevented by the $Ca^{2+}$ agonist verapamil (Fig. 4c) suggesting that AII stimulates $Ca^{2+}$ influx through receptor operated rather than voltage operated channels. The stimulatory effects of isoprenaline and verapamil on renin release were additive (Fig. 2d) suggesting that they operate through different mechanisms. In addition, the finding that BAY K8644, a $Ca^{2+}$ agonist which increases $Ca^{2+}$ influx through potential dependent channels and inhibits renin secretion, does not alter the renin response to isoprenaline (12) suggests that $\beta$-agonists do not alter $Ca^{2+}$ flux through potential dependent channels.

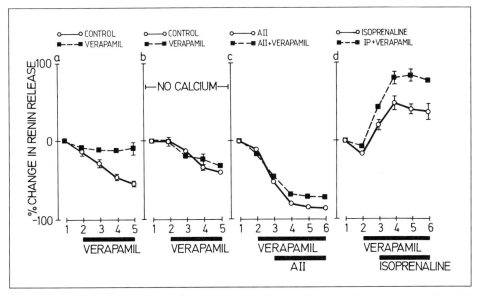

**Fig. 4.** Effect of verapamil ($5 \times 10^{-6}$ M) on basal renin secretion in medium containing 2.5 mM $Ca^{2+}$ (a) and in $Ca^{2+}$ free medium (b). The effect of verapamil on the inhibition of renin secretion by AII ($10^{-5}$ M) (c) and on the stimulation of renin secretion by isoprenaline ($10^{-6}$ M) (d). Means are shown with SEM indicated by a vertical line, except where it is less than the symbol size.

In summary, these studies suggest that the inhibitory effect of AII on basal renin secretion results from increased $Ca^{2+}$ influx causing a rise in intracellular $Ca^{2+}$. However, this mechanism only partially accounts for the inhibition by AII of isoprenaline-stimulated renin secretion. Stimulation of renin secretion by isoprenaline is thought to result from a reduction in intracellular $Ca^{2+}$. This does not result from stimulation of $Na^+/K^+$-ATPase activity leading to $Ca^{2+}$ efflux via $Na^+–Ca^{2+}$ exchange and it is possible that $Ca^{2+}$ efflux via a $Ca^{2+}$-ATPase pump may be the mechanism involved. Movement of $Ca^{2+}$ through potential dependent channels may influence basal renin release but does not appear to be involved in either the inhibition of renin release by AII or the stimulation by isoprenaline. All these findings support the hypothesis that renin release is inversely proportional to intracellular $Ca^{2+}$, but are inferential as levels of intracellular $Ca^{2+}$ were not measured. In a recent report, using a culture containing 80–90% JG cells, AII was shown to cause an increase in intracellular $Ca^{2+}$ as measured by Quin-2 fluorescence (10). This is direct evidence confirming the conclusion that AII inhibits renin secretion by increasing intracellular $Ca^{2+}$.

## Involvement of calmodulin and protein kinase C

These and numerous other studies using kidney slices (3) and isolated kidneys (7) have confirmed the central role that changes in intracellular $Ca^{2+}$ play in the control of renin secretion, but how these changes are coupled to alterations in renin secretion is unclear. The $Ca^{2+}$ binding protein calmodulin, which influences several $Ca^{2+}$ transporting systems, appears to be involved as blockers of calmodulin have been found to stimulate renin secretion (5). Similarly, using our preparation chlorpromazine ($10^{-4}$ M) causes a 150% increase in renin secretion. Other calmodulin blockers have been shown to block the inhibitory effect of $K^+$ depolarisation and high pressure (14) suggesting a role for calmodulin in the inhibition of renin secretion.

Protein kinase C which is activated by diacylglycerol, formed as a result of stimulus evoked hydrolysis of phosphoinositides, is thought to couple receptor occupancy to cell activation. Phorbol esters, which substitute for diacylglycerol and activate protein kinase C, have been shown to enhance $Ca^{2+}$ influx and inhibit renin secretion, suggesting that activation of protein kinase C leads to inhibition of renin secretion (11).

These studies further confirm the hypothesis proposed by Peart that an increase in intracellular $Ca^{2+}$ in the JG cell inhibits renin release, and demonstrate that calmodulin and protein kinase C are probably involved in the secretory process. Further studies are required to determine the mechanisms by which these processes alter $Ca^{2+}$ flux across the membrane, as well as probable release of $Ca^{2+}$ from intracellular stores.

## References

1. Barajas L, Latta H (1967) Structure of the juxtaglomerular apparatus. Circ Res 20 and 21 (Suppl II):15–28
2. Baudouin M, Meyer P, Fermondjian S, Morget J-L (1972) Calcium release induced by interaction of angiotensin with its receptors in smooth muscle cell microsomes. Nature 235:336–338
3. Churchill PC, Churchill MC (1982) Isoproteranol-stimulated renin secretion in the rat: second messenger roles of $Ca^{2+}$ and cyclic AMP. Life Sci. 30 (15):1313–1319
4. Churchill PC, Churchill MC (1982a) $Ca^{2+}$-dependence of the inhibitory effect of $K^+$-depolarization on renin secretion from rat kidney slices. Arch Int Pharmacodyn Ther 258 (2):300–312
5. Churchill PC, Churchill MC (1983) Effects of trifluoperazine on renin secretion of rat kidney slices. J Pharmacol Exp Ther 224 (1):68–72
6. Fray JCS (1980) Mechanism by which renin secretion from perfused rat kidneys is stimulated by isoprenaline and inhibited by high perfusion pressure. J Physiol 308:1–13
7. Fray JCS, Park CS (1979) Influence of potassium, sodium, perfusion pressure and isoprenaline on renin release induced by acute calcium deprivation. J Physiol 292:363–372
8. Fynn M, Onomakpome N, Peart WS (1977) The effects of ionophores (A23187 and RO2-2985) on renin secretion and renal vasoconstriction. Proc R Soc Lond B 199:199–212
9. Hackenthal E, Aktories K, Jacobs KH (1985) Pertussis toxin attenuates angiotensin II-induced vasoconstriction and inhibition of renin release. Mol Cell Endocrinol 42:113–117
10. Kurtz A, Della Bruna R, Pfeilschifter J, Taugner R, Bauer C (1986) Atrial natriuretic peptide inhibits renin release from juxtaglomerular cells by a cGMP-mediated process. Proc Natl Acad Sci 83:4769–4773
11. Kurtz A, Pfeilschifter J, Hutter A, Buhrle C, Nobiling R, Taugner R, Hackenthal E, Bauer C (1986) Role of protein kinase C in inhibition of renin release caused by vasoconstrictors. Am J Physiol 250:C563–C567
12. May CN, Peart WS (1986) Stimulation and suppression of renin release from incubations of rat renal cortex by factors affecting $Ca^{2+}$ flux. Br J Pharmacol 89:173–182
13. Marie J, Gaillard RC, Schoenenberg P, Jard S, Bockaert J (1985) Pharmacological characterization of the angiotensin receptor negatively coupled with adenylate cyclase in rat anterior pituitary gland. Endocrinology 116:1044–1050

14. Park CS, Honeyman TW, Chung ES, Lee JS, Sigmon DH, Fray JCS (1986). Involvement of calmodulin in mediating inhibitory action of intracellular $Ca^{2+}$ on renin secretion. Am J Physiol 251:F1055–F1062
15. Peart WS (1977) The kidney as an endocrine organ. Lancet, ii:543–548
16. Peart WS, Quesada T, Tenyi I (1977) The effects of EDTA and EGTA on renin secretion. Br J Pharmac 59:247–252
17. Van Dongen R, Peart WS (1974). Calcium dependence of the inhibitory effect of angiotensin on renin secretion in the isolation perfused kidney of the rat. Br J Pharmac 50:125–129
18. Woodcock EA, Johnston CI (1982) Inhibition of adenylate cyclase by angiotensin II in rat renal cortex. Endocrinology 111:1687–1691

Authors' address:
Dr. C. N. May,
Medical Unit Laboratory,
St. Mary's Hospital Medical School,
Norfolk Place,
London W2 1PG,
U.K.

# Clinical trials and medical practice

G. Rose

Division of Medical Statistics and Epidemiology, London School of Hygiene and Tropical Medicine, London

This paper will be simpler than others presented at this meeting, and I therefore give it with some diffidence. Several things, nevertheless, give me encouragement. The first is that this is a gathering of friends, in a friendly mood; and that should promote tolerance. The second goes back to an experience soon after I joined the Medical Unit in 1953, when I overheard a patient saying to her husband as she left George Pickering's clinic, "He calls himself a professor, but he couldn't even tell me why I've got high blood pressure!" Listening to today's presentations, I get the impression that things have not changed very much, and an honest doctor would still have to disappoint that lady's expectations.

We have been hearing of Stan Peart's impressive contributions to our under-standing of the mechanisms of hypertension; but he has made equally impressive contributions to the raising of clinical standards through the application of science, combined with good sense, to the care of patients. It was appropriate therefore to include in the programme a paper in recognition of that side of his work.

I have enjoyed the privilege of collaborating with each of our chairmen in a major clinical trial (respectively the MRC [5] and IPPPSH [3] trials), and I offer now a rather arbitrary selection of thoughts arising out of those and other trials of blood pressure management.

## Clinical trials – a changing concept

The original idea of a clinical trial was very simple: it was to answer the question "Does the treatment work?" – to which the true answer was either "Yes" or "No"; the investigator's degree of confidence in his answer was summarised by a P value. A value of 5% distinguished treatments that you should accept from those which could be dumped.

That thinking was current when both the MRC and the IPPPSH trials were set up, and it determined their stopping rules; but it proved quite inadequate to the com-plexities of their results. Part way through the MRC trial we found that treated pa-tients had significantly fewer strokes; so, by our rules, the trial should have stopped. There were however at that time more deaths among treated than control patients, so that to stop at that point would have left the poor clinician thoroughly confused.

At that stage one began to realise that the purpose of a clinical trial is not to test a hypothesis but to guide a clinical decision. This it can best do by estimating the magnitude (with its uncertainty limits) of each major item of benefit and of costs, and assembling the results as a balance-sheet. The clinician and the patient must then judge whether to prefer regime A or B. The trial results should guide that decision, but they do not make it: the decision depends on the values assigned to each of the positive and negative outcomes, and those are a matter for judgement and opinion. No P value, however small, can save doctors the effort of thinking for themselves about their clinical decisions.

This decision-taking approach has so far made little impact on either the planning or reporting of clinical trials. It implies, for example, that a trial should stop, not when a particular outcome reaches some pre-set P-value, but when the results taken as a whole will enable the readers to decide whether they prefer A or B. And it implies that the results need to be expressed in terms of magnitude and confidence interval, not just percentage effects and statistical significance.

## Are selective conclusions appropriate?

That global assessment also proves an oversimplification. If all the MRC trial can tell us is that one stroke could be prevented by 850 patient-years of treatment, perhaps involving 200 years of side-effects, then there might be few takers; but one has to respect the doctor's right to say, "My patient is different!", which leads to a selective application of the results. Indeed, the trial results support that view. The distinguished professor of clinical pharmacology who wrote the BMJ editorial on the MRC trial [5] noted that the percentage reduction in strokes was similar in each of the trial's subgroups; and he concluded that the case for treatment must also be similar, regardless of age. Alas! He confused (as many do) a treatment's proportionate and absolute effects: the latter varied widely (Table 1).

**Table 1.** Estimate from the MRC Hypertension Trial of patient-years of diuretic treatment required to prevent one stroke

| Sex | Age | Smoking | No. of pt-yr |
|-----|-----|---------|--------------|
| M | 60 | + | 100 |
| F | 60 | + | 350 |
| M | 60 | 0 | 500 |
| M | 40 | 0 | 900 |
| F | 40 | 0 | ? |

Since the absolute benefit varies greatly but the side-effects and medical costs are presumably similar in the different categories, it follows that the case for treatment is very different. If you use a particular level of blood pressure as a guide to treatment, then your criterion pressure should be *lower* in men than women, in smokers than non-smokers, and (against the grain!) in older than younger. At the end of the MRC trial we sent a questionnaire to the participating doctors asking about their conclusions on these points. The responses, to put it politely, showed some confusion – particularly on the influence of age and smoking on treatment decisions: most doctors were more ready to treat the younger than the older patients, and many were more hesitant to treat smokers than non-smokers.

To pry in this way among a trial's sub-groups is risky (as we were well aware in both the MRC [5] and IPPPSH [3] trials when we reported an interaction between smoking and benefit from beta-blockers). Some rule it wholly out of court; but that is to suggest that a trial can only tell us whether to treat either all of the patients or none of them. That is not the way that medical practice works, and it is also a waste of trial information. To pry among the sub-groups of a trial is risky, but the hints it yields may be all that we have to go on; and at least they are unbiased. Until something better turns up, it is reasonable that they should guide practice.

## Is normalisation of blood pressure the sole objective?

Doctors tend to see the care of a hypertensive patient as beginning and ending with the normalisation of blood pressure. The sad fact is that normalisation of blood pressure by drugs does little for the patient's main danger, which is from a heart attack. Observational data from both the MRC and IPPPSH trials suggest that a multifactorial approach could be very worthwhile: thus coronary risk was halved among non-smokers, and it was 30% lower for each 10% by which serum cholesterol was lower. To put that multifactorial approach into practice will require some big changes in attitudes and organisation in hypertension clinics, whose attention tends to be confined to control of the blood pressure.

## Non-pharmacological approaches

The thought of treating 10% or 15% of the adult population with antihypertensive drugs seems to be more acceptable in America than Europe. The search for non-pharmacological alternatives has involved mainly weight control, alcohol and salt reduction. Unfortunately no one has yet demonstrated much ability to influence weight or alcohol intake in the long term; and advice on salt reduction has gained popularity more through the lack of alternatives than by positive evidence of its effectiveness. The outcome of Graham Macgregor's elegant trial [4] was positive, but only rather modestly so; and other trials of salt reduction in hypertensives have given little encouragement. As a routine practical therapy, the benefits of advising patients to eat less salt seem scarcely to justify the effort.

Potassium supplementation merits further exploration, as shown by the recent results from a randomised double-blind trial by Mancini's group [6]. But it could be that the critical factor is neither sodium nor potassium as such, but rather some expression of their relationship (in much the same way as the set-point of the hypothalamic temperature-regulating centre apparently depends on the Na/Ca ratio, not the concentration in the cerebrospinal fluid of either individual ion).

To the clinician dealing with an individual patient, a reduction of 3 mmHg in diastolic pressure is unexciting; but a reduction of 3 mmHg in the population average diastolic pressure might save as many lives as the whole of existing antihypertensive medication.

With my colleagues in Portugal we have recently completed a trial of salt reduction in a whole rural community, comparing it with a similar control community. At the outset the daily average adult salt intake was 21 g/day, and 30% of people had a diastolic pressure 95 mmHg or above. Advice on eating less salt was the only intervention. Figure 1 summarises the blood pressure changes. Within the intervention group we also examined the association in individuals between reduction in urinary sodium/creatinine ratio and fall in blood pressure (Table 2). There was a clear tendency for those who most reduced their salt intake also to show the greatest fall in pressure.

This trial shows that in a population eating a great deal of salt the high levels of blood pressure can be substantially reduced by health education, with an expectation of major public health benefits. It does not necessarily indicate what would be achieved by reducing salt intake in the large number of populations consuming around 150–200 mmol of sodium a day.

**Table 2.** Within-subject correlations at one year between change in blood pressure and reduction in urinary sodium/creatinine ratio (Portuguese Salt Trial)

|           | Men    | Women   | Total    |
|-----------|--------|---------|----------|
| Systolic  | +0.13  | +0.27*  | +0.19    |
| Diastolic | +0.11  | +0.37*  | +0.29**  |

$*P<0.05, \ **P<0.02$

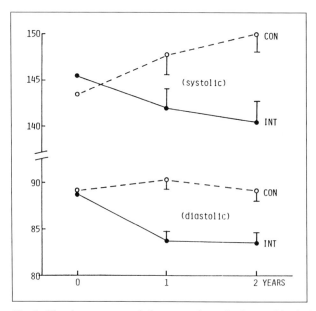

**Fig. 1.** Blood pressure trends (means and standard errors) in the intervention and control communities of the Portugese trial of salt reduction.

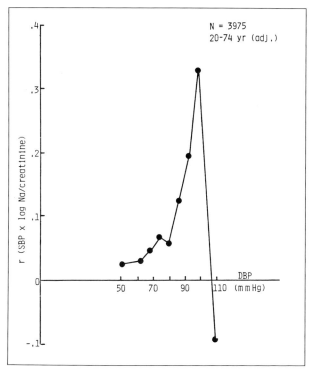

**Fig. 2.** Correlations between diastolic blood pressure and urinary sodium/creatinine ratio in a Brazilian population study, according to level of diastolic pressure [2].

## The salt effect may depend on the pressure

Finally, here is a possible explanation of the discrepant results of the various trials of salt reduction. One of my PhD students, Eduardo Costa, undertook a survey of blood pressure and salt intake in southern Brazil [2]. Figure 2 shows an interesting part of his results, implying not only that the salt/blood pressure relationship may be weak at low levels of blood pressure, but also that at clinically hypertensive levels some other control mechanism may take over. And there rests an ongoing story whose denouement is still to be written.

## Envoi

I owe to George Pickering the origin of a concern to relate clinical trials and epidemiology to the care of hypertension; but it is to Stan Peart that I owe (among other things) the opportunity to implement that concern by working as both epidemiologist and clinician. It has been a good experience, and I am thankful for it.

# References

1. Breckenridge A (1985) Treating mild hypertension. Br Med J 291:89–90
2. Costa E (1981) A cross-sectional survey of blood pressure in Rio Grande do Sul, Brazil – with special reference to salt. London: PhD thesis
3. IPPPSH Collaborative Group (1985) Cardiovascular risk and risk factors in a randomised trial of treatment based on the beta-blocker oxprenolol: the International Prospective Primary Prevention Study in Hypertension (IPPPSH). J Hypertension 3:379–392
4. Macgregor A, Best F, Cam J et al. (1982) Double-blind randomised crossover trial of moderate sodium restriction in essential hypertension. Lancet i:351–355
5. MRC Working Party on Mild to Moderate Hypertension (1985) MRC trial of treatment of mild hypertension: principal results. Br Med J 291:97–104
6. Siani A, Strazzullo P, Russo L et al (1987) Controlled trial of long term oral potassium supplements in patients with mild hypertension. Br Med J 294:1453–1456

Authors' address:
Professor G. Rose
Division of Medical Statistics and Epidemiology
London School of Hygiene and Tropical Medicine
Keppel Street
London, WC1E 7HT

# The genetics of essential hypertension

G. Bianchi*, B. R. Barber**, C. Barlassina*, D. Cusi*, P. Ferrari**,
A. Malavasi, P. Salvati**, S. Salardi**

 * Istituto Scienze Mediche dell'Università degli Studi, Milano;
** Istituto Ricerche Farmitalia Carlo Erba, Nerviano; Milano and
   Istituto di Clinica Medica, Università di Sassari, Italia

## Introduction

The role of genetic factors in essential hypertension is supported by studies of subjects with known genetic relationships (family studies) (41–43) monozygotic twins (25, 26, 37, 38), natural vs adopted children (18) and experimental models of spontaneous or "genetic" hypertension in rats (6, 24, 45). The demonstration that genetic factors are involved in this disease has stimulated many investigators to look for possible biochemical-functional alterations that could be considered as the direct phenotypic expression of genetic abnormalities underlying hypertension. Thus many studies have been performed on human hypertension to investigate alterations of transmembrane ionic transport, intracellular ion content and molecular characteristics of cellular membranes. However, these studies (1, 18, 21, 22, 33, 61) have not resulted in a consistent picture characteristic of the hypertensive patient. This is not surprising considering that essential hypertension is a polygenic disease, phenotypically expressed in different ways depending on the interaction between many environmental factors and a polygenic substrate. When approaching the problem of the etiology of human essential hypertension, it is therefore important to study the same patients with different techniques of physiology, biochemistry, molecular biology and population genetics in order to clarify the sequence of events from genetic alteration to the cellular and organ alteration responsible for the disease in the individual patient or family. Many difficulties hamper this approach in man, the most important being the lack of a theoretical background linking a genetic alteration with a physiological one that may be responsible for hypertension. It could thus be helpful to study an animal model of hypertension, genetically homogeneous. The usefulness of such a model to throw light on the mechanisms underlying human essential hypertension depends on its similarities with the human disease. We have studied the Milan hypertensive strain (MHS) of rats compared with its normotensive control strain (MNS) (9, 14) and humans at the prehypertensive stage (11, 12).

Many experimental observations agree that, to reveal the most characteristic alterations in essential hypertension, it is important to study the early phases of the disease when blood pressure levels are still normal (10). To define a prehypertensive phase in man is more difficult than in rat genetic hypertension. We decided to consider, as prehypertensives, subjects with both parents hypertensive and to compare them with subjects with both parents normotensive. Table 1 shows the similarities found between human prehypertensive subjects and prehypertensive MHS rats compared with their appropriate controls.

**Table 1.** Comparison of prehypertensive humans with rats of the MHS strain

|  | Humans<br>Essential hypertension | Rats<br>MHS |
|---|---|---|
| Pressor effect of the kidney after transplantation | ↑ | ↑ |
| Renal blood flow | ↑ | = |
| GFR | ↑ (+) | ↑ (°) |
| Na excretion after load | ↑ | ↑ |
| 24 h urinary output | ↑ | ↑ |
| Plasma renin | ↓ | ↓ |
| Urine kallikrein | ↓ | ↓ |
| Plasma aldosterone | = | = |
| Plasma Na and K | = | = |
| CO | = | = |

(↑, ↓ = higher, lower or equal in the prehypertensive humans or rats compared to the appropriate controls)
(°) expressed per unit of kidney weight
(+) expressed per unit of body surface area

Both in man (35) and in rats (7) it has been possible to demonstrate, through kidney transplantation experiments, the key involvement of the kidney in the development of hypertension. Kidney function shows the same pattern in man and rats as in their appropriate controls: increased glomerular filtration rate (GFR), 24 h urinary output and Na excretion afterload, with decreased plasma renin activity and urinary kallikrein (8, 11, 12, 28). Renal plasma flow was higher in human predisposed subjects, but similar in predisposed rats compared with controls.

However, recent data on isolated kidney preparations showed that renal vascular resistance is lower in kidneys removed from prehypertensive MHS compared with MNS kidneys (52). No difference was detectable in urine aldosterone or cardiac output in humans. Thus the increase of RPF and GFR seems not to be caused by an abnormality in systemic circulation.

The results reported in the literature on kidney function in offspring of hypertensive parents compared with offspring of normotensive parents are contrasting (3, 20, 34, 41, 53, 55, 63). We discussed this aspect in detail elsewhere (13) and the results published since then (4, 5, 37, 59, 61) have not conflicted with the position expressed in that review.

In view of the reasons given in the introduction, it is not surprising that comparison of the two groups of offspring shows a range of results going from no difference to quite opposite differences, in regard to a given variable, that can be either lower or higher in the predisposed group. If we accept the idea that essential hypertension may originate from different mechanisms, it follows that the renal function pattern may differ in the different predisposed subjects. Why then have we found such a close parallelism between man and rats, since in the latter it is very likely that only one simple genetic mechanism is at work? There are two possible answers to this question.

On is that by chance alone we chose subjects belonging to the same genetic niche where the genetic mechanisms responsible for hypertension were similar to those involved in rat hypertension. In favour of this possibility is the impression (not supported by appropriate statistical analysis because of the insufficient number of subjects) that most predisposed subjects showing the renal function pattern described in Table 1 come from a small town located 50 km north-west of Milan. This group of subjects was reponsible for the shift of the mean of the whole group of predisposed subjects which, on the other hand, included many individual values very similar to those of control subjects (Fig. 1).

The second possibility is that the same major gene effect causes "essential" or genetic hypertension both in man and rats. This is supported by the results so far obtained in hypertensive families (19). In this case the discrepancy among the results of renal function studies mentioned above may also be explained by the low number of subjects for each group of offspring that are clearly insufficient to draw conclusions applicable to the whole population. In fact, the sample sizes in all these studies were clearly less than required for the magnitude of both the standard deviation of the control groups and the difference between the control group and the predisposed group and for the level of error tolerated when concluding that a given difference may or may not really exist and is not due to chance alone (56).

Regardless of which of these two possibilities is true, the only way to approach the problem is that indicated in the introduction, i.e., to link observations at the physiological level with others at the biochemical-molecular level, so that the appropriate tools of molecular biology may be used to assess the responsibility of genetic factors in determining these abnormalities. To procede along these lines it is important to interpret changes in renal function in terms of modification of renal cell function.

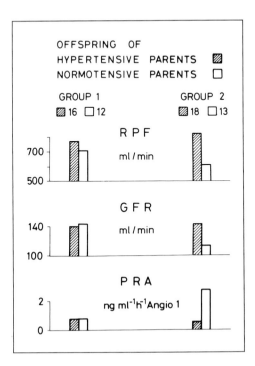

Fig. 1. Differences in renal plasma flow (RPF), glomerular filtration rate (GFR) and plasma renin activity (PRA) in offspring of two hypertensive parents and two normotensive parents, according to the geographical area of origin. Subjects of group 1 were selected in a small town south of Milan (20 km), subjects of group 2 were selected in a small town northeast of Milan (50 km). These results have been already published in (ref. 12) without mentioning the influence of geographical area, because the low number of subjects did not allow appropriate statistical comparisons. It is clear that the typical pattern of changes of the Fam[+] subjects was present only in group 2.

The higher GFR, tubular reabsorption and urinary output, which have also been demonstrated in isolated kidneys (52) removed from prehypertensive MHS rats, may be caused by two mechanisms:

a. An intrinsic abnormality in tubular cell function which causes secondary changes at the glomerular level

b. A primary increase in GFR which is accompanied by secondary changes in tubular cell function.

Micropuncture studies have shown (48, 49) that renal interstitial pressure in prehypertensive MHS is higher than in matched MNS, but this difference disappears within 7–10 days, when a clear difference in blood pressure develops between MHS and MNS and a plasma inhibitor of the Na/K pump increases in MHS (40). Measurements of tubular glomerular feedback sensitivity at these two ages have shown that this sensitivity is lower in MHS at the prehypertensive stage and higher in MHS at the early hypertensive stage (48, 49).

These brusque changes in interstitial hydrostatic pressure and feedback sensitivity may be easily explained by postulating that the primary alteration is a faster tubular reabsorption in MHS which is responsible for both the increased interstitial pressure (which may be involved in the faster excretion of a Na load in MHS) and the development of fluid retention and hypertension.

The increase of renal interstitial pressure may depress the feedback sensitivity, thus leading to a faster GFR (47). When fluid retention triggers the secretion of a factor that inhibits the Na/K pump, tubular reabsorption and renal interstitial pressure will normalize, and, consequently, inhibition of the feedback will be removed. This removal will unmask the greater feedback sensitivity of MHS which is probably due to the genetically determined faster ion transport across the cell membrane of these rats.

This hypothesis must be tested at the cellular level to evaluate whether MHS tubular cells have indeed such a genetically determined faster ion transport across their plasma membrane.

Table 2 summarizes many studies (2, 29, 30, 36, 46, 50, 51, 60) comparing the function of tubular cells of MHS with those of MNS; similar comparisons were also performed on erythrocytes of both strains for reasons that are explained later. It is

**Table 2.** Renal tubular and red blood cell characteristics in MHS (compared with MNS)

|  | Red blood cell | Tubular cell |
|---|---|---|
| Volume | ↓ (30) | ↓ (29) |
| Na content | ↓ (30) | ↓ (2) |
| Na-K cotransport | ↑ (30) | ↑ (*) |
| Na/H countertransport | ? | ↑ (36) |
| Calpain inhibitor (240 kD) | ↓ (50, 51) | ↓ (50, 51) |
| Ca ATPase at $V_{max}$ | ↓ (60) | ↓ (*) |
| $\alpha_2$-receptor density | ? | ↓ (46) |

The arrows indicate greater ( ↑ ) or smaller ( ↓ ) values in MHS rats when compared to MNS rats
Numbers in parentheses refer to publications in which these results are described in detail
(*) refers to unpublished data
? experiments not yet performed

not possible to discuss these studies in detail; however, it is clear that the MHS tubular cells are smaller (29) with less sodium content (2) and faster Na transport across their plasma membrane (36). These differences were detected before the development of hypertension in MHS. However, they may be due to some extracellular factor (either differences in load or humoral) affecting the function of these cells during the period of life preceding these studies.

From Table 2 it is clear that many differences between MHS and MNS in tubular cells are also shared by erythrocytes. Thus the latter cells (which are not affected by any load mechanisms) could be used to establish the responsibility of genetic factors in determining these changes and their possible genetic association with hypertension in hybrids. With bone marrow transplantation (57) from MHS or MNS to F1 hybrids (obtained by crossing MHS with MNS) we demonstrated that the characteristics of the erythrocytes of the two strains could be transplanted, thus the factor(s) responsible for the differences between MHS and MNS was genetically determined within the stem cells. Moreover, in the F2 hybrid populations obtained by crossing the F1 hybrids, the level of blood pressure ranged from the normal value of MNS to the hypertensive values of MHS (57). In this population we found a positive correlation between the rate of erythrocyte Na/K cotransport (one of the abnormalities in Na transport found both in erythrocytes and in tubular cells of MHS) and the levels of blood pressure in the individual rats (15). Therefore, a genetic association between these two traits could be inferred.

In view of the similarities between the erythrocyte and tubular cell abnormalities shown in Table 2, it is very likely that the genetic determination and association with blood pressure demonstrated for one type of cell is also valid for the other type of cell. On the other hand, the role of genetic factors in determining the renal functional characteristics found in MHS was established more than 10 years ago with the demonstration that hypertension can be transferred from MHS to MNS rats by kidney transplantation (7, 32). After having established that a genetically determined abnormality in tubular cells and in erythrocytes was involved in causing hypertension, we approached the problem of identifying which, among the different cellular abnormalities, was primary and genetically determined and which was secondary. In fact, for each mutation compatible with survival of a gene coding for a structural or regulatory protein, in addition to the biochemical abnormality which is the direct phenotypic expression of the mutation, there are other biochemical abnormalities that are caused by readjustment of the overall biochemical machinery of the cell aimed at ensuring a new cellular equilibrium compatible with survival. In both tubular cells and erythrocytes there are differences in cell volume, ion composition, ion transport and protein composition (calpain inhibitor) (see Table 2). Which of these differences is primary? To answer this question we studied erythrocytes of MHS and MNS under different experimental conditions. The results so far obtained are summarized in Table 3. The difference in Na-K cotransport found in intact erythrocytes (15) disappears when this ion transport system is measured in erythrocytes after swelling (when the difference in volume is lost) (30) or in inside-out vesicles (which are membranes deprived of cytoskeleton) (31). Moreover, the difference in cellular volume persists in resealed ghosts which are deprived of intracellular content but still have the membrane cytoskeleton (31). These observations support the notion that the most likely candidate to exert a primary role in determining both

**Table 3.** Red blood cell (RBC) function in MHS (compared to MNS: lower, higher, = equal)

| | |
|---|---|
| a) Volume and Na content in intact RBC | ↓ (30) |
| Volume resealed ghost | ↓ (31) |
| b) Na-K cotransport in intact RBC | ↑ (30) |
| Na-K cotransport (after swelling) | = (30) |
| Na-K cotransport in inside-out vesicles | = (31) |
| (deprived of cytoskeleton) | |

Results obtained by studying erythrocytes in different experimental conditions (↑, ↓, = higher, lower or equal in MHS compared to MNS rats)
Numbers in parentheses refer to publications in which these results are described in detail

the differences in volume and Na-K cotransport between MHS and MNS is located within the network of proteins that form the membrane cytoskeleton. To test this hypothesis, we injected ghosts or membrane cytoskeleton of MHS or MNS into both animals of the same or of the other strain with the aim of discovering a difference between MHS and MNS in the antigenic structure of one of the cytoskeleton proteins. The most constant result in these experiments was the formation of an antibody against a 105 KDa cytoskeleton protein when MHS rats were immunized with MNS cell membrane (27). The details of the experiments that followed this observation are described elsewhere (54) and can be briefly described as follows: the antibody against the 105 KDa protein was used to screen a cDNA library of mouse erythroid tissue and to select a clone producing a 31 KDa protein which is recognized by the antibody (54). Rabbits immunized with the 31 KDa protein form an antibody which recognizes the 105 KDa natural protein in a very selective way. The sequence of the insert (the DNA coding for the 31 KDa protein) has been determined and it does not correspond to any known protein so far sequenced.

Studies are in progress to isolate the complete sequence of the gene coding for the whole 105 KDa protein. Preliminary unpublished studies carried out on this protein have shown very interesting functional characteristics. The 105 KDa protein binds phosphatidylserine, calmodulin and protein kinase C and is phosphorylated by the kinase. The binding activity is reduced when the protein is phosphorylated. These functional characteristics suggest that this protein may have a role in the binding of the membrane cytoskeleton to the lipid bilayer of the cell membrane and it may also have a function in the crosslinking of the other cytoskeleton proteins. Therefore, an abnormal function of this protein may, theoretically, account for abnormalities in the regulation of cell volume and ion transport across the cell membrane.


**Cell function in human essential hypertension**

Based on the above results, we studied Na transport across erythrocyte membrane with the aim of verifying if, as in rats, ion transport systems in man are under genetic control and are in someway related to hypertension. Although the results in rats justified the use of the red blood cell as a tubular cell model, we wanted to see whether a link between ion transport in erythrocytes and proximal tubular function could also be found in man.

The degree of genetic influence on ion transports and Na content were investigated by analyzing the correlations between spouses and between offspring and parents in families with a different history of hypertension.

Our data show that Na content and Na pump of red blood cells are mainly influenced by the environment because they correlate significantly between spouses, whereas Na-K cotransport and Na-Li countertransport are not (22). For Na-Li countertransport, on the contrary, a close correlation was observed between parents and offspring in both normotensive and hypertensive families, whereas for Na-K cotransport a correlation was found only in the hypertensive families (23).

This last observation could depend on a greater genetic polymorphism of this character in the hypertensive population, which may well be secondary to a dominant mutation of a gene coding for a protein, like the rat 105 KDa protein, that may have a regulatory function on Na-K cotransport.

Our second objective was to find a correlation between erythrocyte and tubular cell function and to investigate the possibility of an increased proximal tubular reabsorption. We found that both Na-K cotransport and Na-Li countertransport correlate inversely with fractional excretion of uric acid, and Na-Li countertransport correlates positively with renal reabsorption of lithium (23) (which may be considered a marker of proximal tubular reabsorption (58). This indicates that patients with high Na-K cotransport and Na-Li countertransport may have an increased proximal reabsorption.

## Future directions

If the sequence of events from gene abnormality to renal functional abnormality discussed for MHS rats proves to be true, then we shall have some tools to study the role of erythrocytes and renal functional abnormalities in the pathogenesis of essential hypertension. In fact, the antibody against the rat 105 KDa protein also recognizes a 105 KDa protein in urine and human erythrocytes as well other proteins in the brain and renal tissues of rats.

The following measurements should be performed in the individual members of hypertensive families:
1. Polymorphism of the DNA region coding for the 105 KDa protein
2. Function of the 105 KDa protein as regards its ability to phosphorylate after binding to protein kinase C, and its ability to bind calmodulin and phosphatidylserine under specific experimental conditions
3. Functional characteristics of the erythrocytes (volume, sodium content, ion transports, etc)
4. Functional characteristics of the kidneys
5. Level of blood pressure under different environmental circumstances.

Only in this way can we circumvent the problems arising from polygenic inheritance and interaction of a given gene abnormality with different genetic backgrounds and with different environmental factors.

Using this approach we might be able to show that one of the mechanisms leading to essential hypertension in man operates through a sequence of events similar to that of MHS. The many similarities between MHS and humans at the prehypertensive stage, shown above, justify this study in humans.

## References

1. Ambrosioni E, Costa FV, Montebugnoli L, Borghi C, Vasconi L, Tartagni F. Magnani B (1981) Intralymphocytic sodium concentration. A sensitive index to identify young subjects at risk of hypertension. Clin Exp Hypertens 3:675–691
2. Beck F, Bianchi G, Dorge A, Rick R, Schramm M, Thurau K (1983) Sodium and potassium concentrations of renal cortical cells in two animal models of primary arterial hypertension. J Hypertension 1 (Suppl 2):38–39
3. Baldwin DS, Biggs AW, Goldring W, Hulet WH, Chasis H (1958) Exaggerated natriuresis in essential hypertension. Am J Med 24:893–902
4. Bianchetti MG, Beretta-Piccoli C, Weidman P, Ferrier C (1986) Blood pressure control in normotensive members of hypertensive families. Kidney Int 29:882–888
5. Bianchetti MG, Weidman P, Beretta-Piccoli C, Ferrier C (1987) Potassium and norepinephrine or angiotensin mediated pressor control in pre-hypertension. Kidney Int 31:956–963
6. Bianchi G, Fox U (1974) The development of a new strain of spontaneously hypertensive rats. Life Sci 14:339–347
7. Bianchi G, Fox U, Di Francesco GF, Bardi U, Radice M (1974) Blood pressure changes produced by kidney cross-transplantation between spontaneously hypertensive rats and normotensive rats. Clin Sci Mol Med 47:435–448
8. Bianchi G, Baer PG, Fox U, Duzzi L, Pagetti D, Giovannetti AM (1975) Changes in renin, water balance and sodium balance during development of high blood pressure in genetically hypertensive rats. Circ Res 36 & 37 (Suppl 1):I-153/I-161
9. Bianchi G, Baer PG (1976) Characteristics on the Milan hypertensive strain (MHS) of rats. Clin Exp Pharmacol Physiol (Suppl 3):15–20
10. Bianchi G, Baer PG, Fox U, Guidi E (1977) The role of the kidney in the rat with genetic hypertension. Post Grad Med J 53 (Suppl 2):123–125
11. Bianchi G, Cusi D, Gatti M, Lupi P, Ferrari P, Barlassina C, Picotti GB, Colombo G, Gori D, Velis O, Mazzei D (1979) A renal abnormality as a possible cause of essential hypertension. Lancet I:173–175
12. Bianchi G, Cusi D, Barlassina C, Lupi P, Ferrari P, Picotti GB, Gatti M, Polli E (1983) Renal dysfunction as a possible cause of essential hypertension in predisposed subjects. Kidney Int 23:870–875
13. Bianchi G, Barlassina C (1983) Renal function in essential hypertension. In: Genest J, Kuchel O, Hamet P, Cantin M (eds) Hypertension: Physiopathology and treatment. McGraw Hill, New York, p 54–73
14. Bianchi G, Ferrari P, Barber BR (1984) The Milan Hypertension strain. de Jong W (ed) Handbook of hypertension Vol 4: Experimental and genetic models of hypertension. Elsevier Science B.V., pp 328–349
15. Bianchi G, Ferrari P, Trizio D, Ferrandi M, Torielli L, Barber BR, Polli E (1985) Red blood cell abnormalities and spontaneous hypertension in the rat. A genetically determined link. Hypertension 7:319–329
16. Bianchi G, Barber BR, Ferrari P, Duzzi L (1987) The Milan hypertensive strain of rats and its controls normotensive strain. Hypertension 9 (Suppl I):I-30/I-33
17. Biron P, Mongeau JG, Bertrand D (1976) Familial aggregation of blood pressure in 558 adopted children. Can Med Assoc J 115:773–774
18. Canessa M, Adragna N, Solomon HS, Connolly TM, Tosteson DC (1980) Increased sodium-lithium countertransport in red cells of patients with essential hypertension. New Engl J Med 302:772–776
19. Cavalli Sforza L, Bodmer WF. In: The genetics of human populations 2. W. H. Freeman & Co, San Francisco
20. Cottier PT, Weller JM, Hoobler SW (1958) Effect of intravenous sodium chloride load on renal haemodynamics and electrolyte excretion in essential hypertension. Circulation 17:750–760
21. Cusi D, Barlassina C, Ferrandi M, Palazzi P, Celega E, Bianchi G (1981) Relationship between altered Na-K cotransport and Na-Li countertransport in the erythrocytes of essential hypertensive patients. Clin Sci 61 (Suppl):33s–36s
22. Cusi D, Tripodi G, Alberghini E, Niutta E, Barlassina C, Fossali E, Dossi F, Bianchi G (1986) Heritability of sodium transport systems and hypertension. Bianchi G, Carafoli E, Scarpa A (eds) Ann N Y Acad Sci Vol 488, pp 576–578

23. Cusi D, Barlassina C, Tripodi G, Niutta E, Alberghini E, Pozzoli E, Pati P, Dossi F, Colombo R, Fassali E, Bianchi G (1987) Genetic factors in ion transport abnormalities in essential hypertension. J Hypertension 5 (Suppl 5)

24. Dahl LK, Heine M, Tassinari L (1962) Role of genetic factors in susceptibility to experimental hypertension due to chronic excess salt ingestion. Nature 194:480–482

25. Feinleib M, Garrison R, Borhani N, Rosenman R, Christian J (1975) In: Paul O (ed) Studies of hypertension in twins, in epidemiology and control of hypertension. Stratten, New York, pp 3–17

26. Feinleib M, Garrison RJ, Fabsitz R, Christian JC, Hrubec Z, Borhani NO (1977) The NHLBI twin study of cardiovascular disease risk factors: methodology and summary of results. Am J Epidemiol 106:284–295

27. Ferrandi M, Salardi S, Modica R, Bianchi G (1987) Antigenic Properties of erythrocyte membrane from a hypertensive strain of rats. In: Bianchi G, Carafoli E, Scarpa A (eds) Endocytobiology III Vol 503, pp 584–587

28. Ferrari P, Cusi D. Barber BR, Barlassina C, Vezzoli G, Duzzi L, Minotti E, Bianchi G (1982) Erythrocyte membrane and renal function in relation to hypertension in rats of the Milan hypertensive strain. Clin Sci 63:61s–63s

29. Ferrari P, Nussdorfer G, Torielli L, Salvati P, Tripodi MG, Niutta E, Bianchi G (1986) Renal function and cell characteristics during the development of essential and genetic hypertension. In: Early Pathogenesis of primary Hypertension – proceedings of the International Symposium, Rotterdam, Elsevier Science Publishers BV

30. Ferrari P, Ferrandi M, Torielli L, Canessa M, Bianchi G (1987) Relationship between erythrocyte volume and sodium transport in the Milan hypertensive rat and age dependent changes. J Hypertension 5:199–206

31. Ferrari P, Torielli L, Ferrandi M, Cirillo M, Bianchi G (1986) Volumes and $Na^+$ transports in intact red blood cells, resealed ghosts and inside-out vesicles of Milan hypertensive rats. J Hypertension 4 (Suppl 6):S379–S381

32. Fox U, Bianchi G (1976) The primary role of the kidney in causing the blood pressure differences between the Milan hypertensive strain (MHS) and normotensive rats. Clin Exp Pharmacol Physiol Suppl 3:71–74

33. Garay RP, Meyer P (1979) A new test showing abnormal net Na and K fluxes in erythrocytes of essential hypertensive patients. Lancet I:349–353

34. Grim CE, Luft FC, Miller JZ, Rose RJ, Christian JC, Weinberger MH (1980) An approach to the valutation of genetic influences on factors that regulate arterial blood pressure in man. Hypertension 2 (Suppl 1):I-34/I-42

35. Guidi E, Bianchi G, Dallosta C, Cantaluppi A, Mandelli V, Vallino F, Polli E (1982) The influence of familial hypertension of the donor on the blood pressure and antihypertensive therapy of kidney graft recipients. Nephron 30:318–323

36. Hanozet G, Parenti P, Salvati S (1985) Presence of a potential-sensitive $Na^+$ transport across renal brush-border membrane vesicles from rats of the Milan hypertensive strain. Biochem Biophys Acta 819:179–186

37. Harvard B, Haage M (1965) Hereditary factors elucidated by twin studies, in genetics and the epidemiology of chronic disease. In: Neel JV, Shaw MW, Schull WJ (eds) Publication 1163, U.S. Department of Health, Education and Welfare, Public Health Service, Washington

38. Havlik RJ, Garrison RJ, Katz SH, Ellison RC, Feinleib M (1979) Detection of genetic variance in blood pressure of seven-year old twins. Am J Epidemiol 109:512–516

39. Hohn AR, Riopelle DA, Keill JE, Loadholt CB, Margolius HS, Halushka PV, Privitera PJ, Webb JG, Medley ES, Schumann SH, Rubin MI, Pantel RH, Braunstein ML (1983) Childhood familial and racial differences in physiologic and biochemical factors related to hypertension. Hypertension 5:56–69

40. Holland S, Millet J, Alaghband-Zadeh J, de Wardener H, Ferrari P, Bianchi G (1987) Cytochemically assayable Na-K ATPase inhibition by Milan hypertensive rat plasma. Hypertension 9:498–503

41. Hollenberg NK, Williams GH, Adams DF (1981) Essential hypertension: abnormal renal vascular and endocrine responses to a mild physiological stimulus. Hypertension 3:11–17

42. Mial WE, Oldham (1958) Factor influencing arterial blood pressure in the general population. Clin Sci 17:409

43. Miall WE (1959) Follow-up study of arterial pressure in the population of a welsh mining valley. Brit Med J 2:1204–1210
44. Miall WE, Heneage P, Khosal T, Lovell HG, Morre F (1967) Factors influencing the degree of resemblance in arterial pressure of closer relatives. Clin Sci 33:271–283
45. Okamoto K, Aoki K (1963) Development of a strain of spotaneously hypertensive rats. Jpn Circ J 27:282–293
46. Parini A, Diop L, Ferrari P, Bondiolotti GP, Dausse JP, Bianchi G (1987) Selective modification of renal alpha-2 adrenoceptors in Milan hypertensive rat strain. Hypertension (in press)
47. Persson AEG, Boberg U, Hahne B, Muller-Suur, Norlen BJ, Selen G (1982) Interstitial pressure as a modulator of tubulo-glomerular feed-back control. Kidney Int 22:12–128
48. Persson AEG, Bianchi G, Boberg U (1984) Evidence of defective tubulo-glomerular feed-back control in rats of the Milan hypertensive strain (MHS). Acta Physiol Scand 122:217–219
49. Persson AEG, Bianchi G, Boberg U (1985) Tubuloglomerular feedback in hypertensive rats of the Milan strain. Acta Physiol Sand 123:139–146
50. Pontremoli S, Melloni E (1986) Decreased level of calpain inhibitor activity in red blood cells from Milan hypertensive rats. Biochem Biophys Res Commun 138 (3):1370–1375
51. Pontremoli S, Melloni E, Salamino F, Sparatore B, Michetti M, Sacco O, Bianchi G (1987) Characterization of the defective calpain-endogenous calpain inhibitor system in erythrocytes from Milan hypertensive rats. Biochem Biophys Res Commun 145 (3):1287–1294
52. Salvati P, Pinciroli GP, Bianchi G (1984) Renal function of isolated perfused kidneys from hypertensive (MHS) and normotensive (MNS) rats of the Milan strain at different ages. J Hypertension 2 (Suppl 3):351–353
53. Schalekamp MADH, Krass XH, Schalekam-Kuyken MPA, Kolsters G, Birkenhager WH (1971) Studies on the mechanisms of hypernatriuresis in essential hypertension in relation to measurements of plasma renin concentration, body fluid compartments and renal function. Clin Sci 41:219–231
54. Sidoli et al.: in preparation
55. Statius Van Eps LW, Birkenhager WH, Stertefeld T (1962) The involved van de lichaamshouding op de "hipernatriuresis" bij lijders aan hypertensive (the influence of posture on hypernatriuresis in hypertensive patients). Ned Tijdshr Geneesk 106:623–628
56. Stolley PD, Strom BL (1986) Sample size calculations for clinical pharmacology studies. Clin Pharmacol Ther 39:489–490
57. Trizio D, Ferrari P, Ferrandi M, Torielli L, Bianchi G (1983) Expression at the hemopoietic stem cell level of the genetically determined erythrocyte membrane defects in the Milan hypertensive rat strain (MHS). J Hypertension 1 (Suppl 2):6–8
58. Thomsen K, Schou Ma (1968) Renal lithium excretion in man. Am J Physiol 154:823–827
59. Uneda S, Fujishima S, Fujiki Y, Tochikubo O, Oda H, Asahina S, Kanedo Y (1984) Renal haemodynamics and the renin-angiotensin system in adolescents genetically predisposed to essential hypertension. J Hypertension (Suppl 3):437–439
60. Vezzoli G, Elli A, Tripodi MG, Bianchi G, Carafoli E (1985) Calcium ATPase in erythrocytes of spontaneously hypertensive rats of the Milan strain. J Hypertension 3:645–648
61. Watt GCM, Foy CJW, Hart BJT (1983) Comparison of blood pressure, sodium intake and other variables in offspring with and without a family history of high blood pressure. Lancet I:1245–1248
62. Wessel (1980) Intracellular electrolytes and arterial hypertension. In: Zumkley, Losse
63. Wiggins RC, Basar I, Slater JDH (1978) Effect of arterial pressure and inheritance on the sodium excretory capacity of normal young man. Clin Sci Mol Med 54:639–647

Authors' address:
G. Bianchi,
Istituto Scienze Mediche,
dell'Università degli Studi,
Milano, Italia

# Migration studies and blood pressure: A model for essential hypertension

P. S. Sever, N. R. Poulter, K. T. Khaw

Department of Clinical Pharmacology, St. Mary's Hospital Medical School, London, UK

## Introduction

Studies of experimental animals and man have provided evidence that both environmental and genetic factors are important determinants of arterial pressure. Whilst much information has been gained from detailed investigations of experimental models of hypertension, the direct applicability of such studies to the aetiology and pathogenesis of essential hypertension in man is by no means clear, and what is needed is an appropriate human model of the hypertensive process. Cross-sectional studies have demonstrated that rural/urban migration, particularly of individuals migrating from an unacculturated society to an urban environment, is frequently associated with a rise in blood pressure, and we have considered the possibility that this process might be such a model. We suggest that the factors involved in the rise in blood pressure with migration, be they genetic or environmental, are the same factors responsible for the rise in blood pressure with age seen in westernised societies, and also the factors responsible for the pathogenesis of essential hypertension (Fig. 1).

Towards the end of the 1970s a reappraisal was taking place of the direction of research carried out at the Wellcome Trust Research Laboratories in Nairobi. For decades the Unit had devoted its attention to research into "tropical" diseases such as anaemia and schistosomiasis. However, the Trust decided upon a change of direction in order to support a programme of cardiovascular research which would include studies designed to further investigate the role of environmental factors in the aetiology and pathogenesis of high blood pressure. Opportunity was therefore taken in collaboration with the Kenya Medical Research Institute, to study the effects on blood pressure of rural-urban migration in a remote Kenyan group of the Luo tribe.

Initially cross-sectional studies of blood pressure were conducted in an attempt to identify a rural population in which blood pressures were low and rose little with age. In the first population studied, which was superficially unacculturated, an age- blood pressure relationship which resembled that encountered in urban or westernised environments was found. Closer observations of this group revealed that many "western" influences, including the use of packaged and processed foods, had already been introduced into this society and consequently it was necessary to cast the net further afield to a group of Luo tribes people in Western Kenya in order to find a group where blood pressures were low and failed to rise with age. On discovering such a community (studies on which we have previously reported, [1, 2], we traced and studied all those residents of Kenya's capital city, Nairobi, who originated from

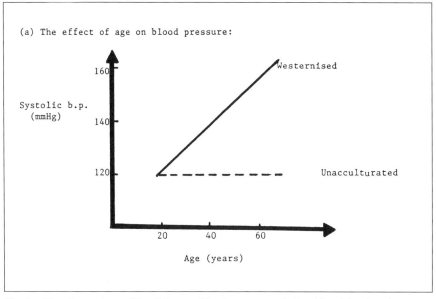

**Fig. 1 a.** The change in profile of the age-blood pressure relationship with migration.

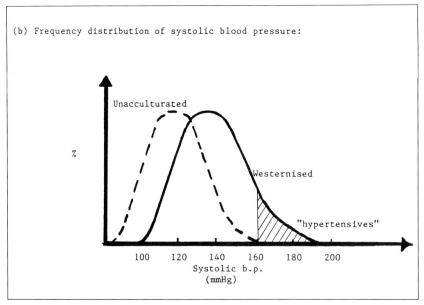

**Fig. 1 b.** Frequency distribution of blood pressure in an unacculturated population and the shift to the right of the curve in urban migrants.

this low blood pressure community to confirm that their blood pressures were significantly higher than their rural counterparts and rose more steeply with age. This having been achieved, a unique longitudinal migration study was initiated in order to determine the rate at which blood pressure changes with migration, the magnitude of the blood pressure rise and the possible factors responsible for the change in arterial pressure.

It is on the basis of the early results from this study that the present hypothesis was evolved.

## The longitudinal study

Details of the methodology involved in the longitudinal study are described else-where [3]. In brief, over 380 new migrants to Nairobi from the low blood pressure rural community in western Kenya, were investigated very shortly after arrival in Nairobi, and thereafter at 3, 6, 12, 18 and 24 months following migration. A cohort of age, sex and geographically-matched rural-based controls were studied under identical conditions. Results obtained from an early analysis of the data for the first six months of follow-up (Fig. 2) clearly demonstrated both weight and urinary electrolyte (Na/K) ratio to be significantly and independently correlated

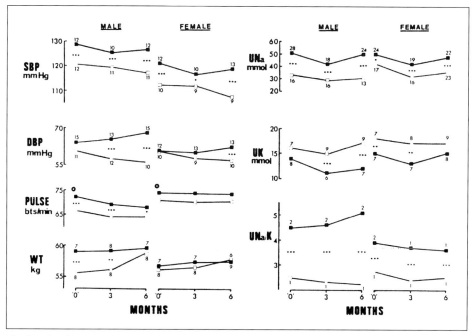

Fig. 2. Blood pressure (SBP, systolic: DBP, diastolic), pulse rate, body weight (WT), mean of three 12 h overnight urine sodium (UNa), potassium (UK) and Na/K ratio (UNa/K) in migrants (male n = 78, female n = 61) and controls (male n = 126, female n = 78) during six months' follow-up. Figures in parentheses are standard deviations of the mean; * p < 0.05; ** p < 0.01; *** p < 0.001. Age-adjusted values using analysis of variance, therefore no s.d. for pulse rates.

with the blood pressure differences between the migrants and the controls. Moreover, early changes in systolic pressure were related to the differences in pulse rate [3].

From this analysis we suggested that the relationship to pulse implied that an autonomic mechanism, perhaps stress induced, might be causally related to some of the blood pressure rise with migration, although this effect was largely confined to systolic pressure and decreased with time. It was also evident from the analyses that both weight change and an increase in dietary sodium, accompanied by a decrease in dietary potassium, as reflected by urinary electrolyte analyses, were determinants of a proportion of the blood pressure rise.

## Environmental changes with migration

The nature and the magnitude of changes occurring with migration or acculturation will inevitably vary with each migrating population. However, for rural/urban migrants, acculturation consists of exposure to a new and challenging environment at a time when there are also important changes in their diets. Dietary histories and analyses of individual diets of this migrating population suggest that migration is associated with an increase in dietary sodium, a reduction in potassium and an increase in the intake of processed foods and refined carbohydrates (Poulter et al., unpublished data). Animal protein intake is increased, there is a reduction in vegetable protein and there is an increase in the intake of all forms of fat. Unlike most other rural-urban migrant data, in this particular study there was no apparent initial increase in total caloric intake. The quantitative determinations of urinary electrolytes in multiple 12- or 24-h urine samples have provided some clues to the magnitude of the change in dietary sodium and potassium and, although the increase in sodium intake is relatively small, it is compatible with a dietary salt hypothesis. It may be that the absolute increase in sodium, from an average of 60 mmols to 100 + mmols of sodium per day, may well constitute a change across a concentration range of greater relevance to blood pressure than similar increases of 40–50 mmol per day occurring in a westernised society that regularly consumes very much larger quantities, (of the order of 150–200 mmol) per day [4]. The reduction in dietary potassium and the consequent increase in urinary Na/K ratio is also compatible with the view that dietary potassium may have an independent inverse relationship to blood pressure.

In addition to the major changes in diet, we believe that the phenomenon of acculturation is expressed in physiological terms by a defence reaction and that environmental stress operating through limbic-hypothalamic pathways may maintain or increase sympathetic outflow primarily to the heart and the kidneys at a time when individual migrants are exposed to increases in dietary sodium and that this neurogenic factor may markedly influence the normal homeostatic response to the dietary sodium load.

The normal physiological response to a sudden increase in dietary sodium has been extensively investigated. The primary neurogenic response would result from the rise in cardiopulmonary blood volume in response to salt loading, causing stimulation of central low pressure volume receptors and negative feedback inhibition of sympathetic outflow, particularly to the heart and kidneys. The reduction in renal sympathetic efferent nerve traffic, with its resultant effects on the renal vasculature and, perhaps more importantly, on the renal tubular handling of sodium, would lead to a reduction in sodium reabsorption and a natriuresis (Fig. 3a). Other factors contribute to the homeostatic response to salt loading, including suppression of the renin-angiotensin-aldosterone system facilitating the renal excretion of the excess sodium load, and the release of atrial natriuretic hormone, occurring in response to atrial wall stretch, consequent upon the rise in cardiopulmonary blood volume. Any blood pressure response to this degree of sodium loading, whether explained by autoregulation or by the release of a natriuretic hormone with vasopressor characteristics, one would predict would be small, at least initially, and could not simply explain the magnitude of the rise in blood pressure we have observed in many of the Luo migrants.

One therefore has to seek an additional explanation for the early pressure rise, which would, perhaps in part, involve a modest increase in dietary sodium. One slightly puzzling observation in the early days following migration was the dramatic increase in body weight of the order of 2 kilos which we felt was unlikely to be related to an overall increase in total caloric intake, since this seemed improbable from our estimates based on dietary histories and food analyses. A more probable explanation was that the weight increase represented an early period of sodium and water retention and that the normal homeostatic response to sodium loading had in some way been modified or prevented.

The hypothesis proposed therefore is an interaction of the response of the autonomic nervous system to the environmental stress of migration with a sudden increase in dietary sodium. The increased sympathetic outflow, primary to the heart and kidneys, occurring as part of the defence reaction overrides the negative feedback inhibition of renal sympathetic nerve activity which would normally be expected with sodium loading. Hence the kidney retains sodium and water and a volume dependent rise in blood pressure occurs initially (Fig. 3b). A further mechanism which would facilitate sodium and water retention in migrants and which would occur as part of the stress response would be a glucocorticoid effect consequent upon the hypothalamic release of ACTH. Measurements of corticosteroid responses to the migration phenomenon have, however, not been undertaken in this study.

The relationship between stress and blood pressure is difficult to evaluate critically. There is no doubt that acute stresses of a mental or physical nature can have immediate effects on blood pressure and autonomic mechanisms are clearly involved, however, the longer term effects of stress on blood pressure have been hard to establish, essentially because of the difficulty in defining and quantifying environmental stress. However, it is interesting to note from recent studies in which blood pressure has been more carefully analysed by means of 24-h ambulatory blood pressure recordings, that work and environmental stress may have more prolonged influences upon blood pressure than had hitherto been perceived by means of conventional clinical blood pressure recordings [5].

It is tempting to extrapolate to humans from animal models of experimental hypertension, such as the spontaneously hypertensive rat (SHR), in which 'stress' appears to play an aetiological role in blood pressure elevation – but supporting

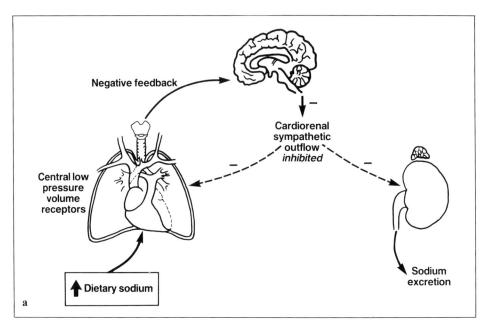

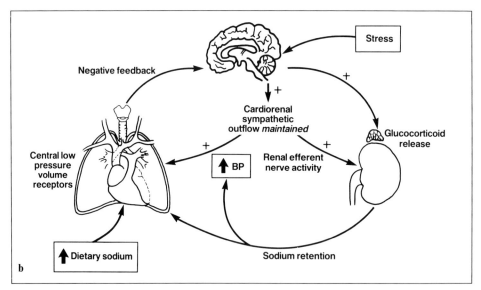

**Figs. 3a, b.** Possible mechanisms involved in the early blood pressure response to migration. Fig. 3a shows the normal physiological response to sodium loading with an increase in central blood volume triggering the low pressure receptors leading to negative feedback inhibition of cardiorenal sympathetic outflow and the facilitation of sodium excretion. Figure 3b shows the basis for the hypothesis, where cardiorenal sympathetic outflow is maintained or increased in response to environmental stress and overrides the negative feedback inhibition of sympathetic outflow normally associated with the sodium load. The hypothesis demands that both stress *and* dietary sodium are implicated in the blood pressure elevation. At least some of the variation in individual response may be determined by genetic abnormality in the kidney, facilitating sodium reabsorption in response to stress.

evidence is scarce. Evidence from the Tolekau Island migrant study supports the hypothesis that some functions of acculturation amongst migrants from an isolated community to an urbanised society of different ethnic backgrounds is associated with an increase in blood pressure [6]. In this study, some attempt was made to quantify the degree of acculturation and it was found to correlate positively with blood pressure.

No analysis of acculturation is available on the Kenyan migrants, but the constellation of challenges imposed on new migrants, such as different housing, exposure to people of different tribes, languages and dialects, the uncertainties of day to day urban and suburban living and their inherent violence, undoubtedly represent great environmental stresses. It is regrettable that no simple, measurable and reproducible determinants of such environmental stress can be incorporated in studies of this nature.

The interaction between the sympathetic nervous system and dietary sodium has received attention in recent years, particularly in various animal models of essential hypertension. The development of hypertension in the SHR is associated with increased renal retention of sodium [7]. Recent studies have shown that environmental stress exacerbates hypertension in the SHR [8] and the addition of increased dietary sodium intake to the environmental stress in the SHR further exacerbates the hypertension [9]. In sodium or volume dependent models of hypertension in the rat such as 1K Goldblatt hypertension or DOCA salt hypertension, there is evidence that the sympathetic nervous system plays a role in maintaining the blood pressure rise [10, 11]. Also in the DOCA salt model environmental stress enhances the degree of sodium retention by increasing renal efferent sympathetic nerve activity and tubular reabsorption of sodium [12].

It seems possible, therefore, that these experimental forms of hypertension may have their parallel in the human model described in this paper. Migrants increase their dietary sodium intake at a time when they are simultaneously exposed to environmental stress resulting in increased renal nerve activity, sodium and water retention and an increase in blood pressure.

Although no detailed analysis of the diets in the Kenyan study is yet available, it is possible that other changes in dietary constituents could contribute to sympathetic outflow and to sodium and water retention. Of particular interest is the increase in intake of refined carbohydrates which may be associated with increased sympathetic activity, insulin secretion and salt and water retention [13, 14]. If any such mechanisms were operative in migrants, the effects would be additive to those imposed by environmental stress and an increase in dietary salt.


**Individual responses to migration**

So far we have only discussed the group mean data derived from the migration study. Obviously individual responses vary and in the following figure (Fig. 4) information is shown on the early systolic blood pressure responses to migration. It should be emphasised that these changes in individual blood pressures occurred during a mean migration time of four weeks with a range of 1–60 days. For the group as a whole the mean increase in systolic pressure is 9.5 mmHg and the range +36 to

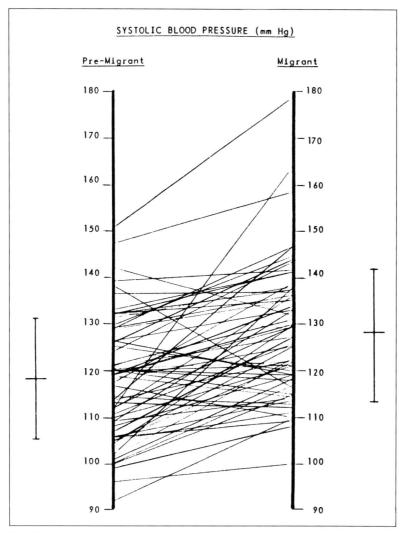

**Fig. 4.** Systolic blood pressures obtained in individuals in the rural community and their corresponding values obtained shortly after migration (an average of four weeks). Mean values ± 1 SD are also shown.

−22 mmHg. Of particular importance is the fact that the distribution of these changes is unimodal and hence there is no suggestion of bimodality which would imply a sensitive or resistant subgroup. We believe that the explanation of these individual differences in blood pressure responses to migration reflects not only quantum differences in the environmental stimulus, but also a variable genetic predisposition to cope with change, and we would speculate that the rise in blood pressure reflects a failure of adaptation to the new environment, more specifically a failure of homeostatic mechanisms to respond to the varying perturbations of the cardiovascular system that have been initated by the urbanisation process.

The anthropologist Scotch hypothesised that high blood pressures resulted from the failure of the individual to meet the demands of a changing environment with adaptive behaviour [15]. His view was amplified by Cruz-Coke who suggested that unacculturated populations may enjoy an unchallenging and unchanging tradition over generations and when their ecological niche is breached and there is cultural change, lack of adaptation of some individuals may be the initiating factor in the pathogenesis of their blood pressure rise [16]. This in the context of an increased sodium load may apply to our Luo migrants in Kenya.

The site at which an underlying genetic abnormality which predisposes certain individuals to blood pressure elevation with migration remains, of course, uncertain. That genetic factors may play a major part in determining the physiological responses to the combined environmental effects of stress and dietary sodium loading, is evident from a number of experimental models of hypertension. For example, in the spontaneously hypertensive rat, environmental stress is associated with an increase in renal efferent sympathetic nerve activity and antinatriuresis. This response is enhanced by sodium loading. On the other hand, in the Wistar Kyoto control animals, the combined effects of stress and salt loading produce no such effect [9]. It is possible that the genetic predisposition in the spontaneously hypertensive rat is located in the central nervous system and that these animals are hyper-responsive to environmental stress, particularly since high sodium intake in these animals may also increase the sensitivity of the hypothalamus to electrical stimuli which in turn result in increased sympathetic outflow [17].

On the other hand, there is evidence that the kidney is the more likely site for the genetic "lesion" in many experimental models. For example, in the cross-transplantation studies of Bianchi [18], the role of the kidney in the pathogenesis of hypertension in the spontaneously hypertensive rat was confirmed. More recently Bianchi has demonstrated that in man the use of drugs to control blood pressure after renal transplantation is greater in recipients of transplants from donors who had a family history of hypertension compared with those who came from normotensive families [19].

The interrelationship of stress and sodium and the effects of familial factors in man has rarely been studied. In one study, a stressful competitive task produced an anti-natriuretic response only in subjects with a positive family history of hypertension and not in those with normotensive parents [20]. We are currently in the process of repeating and extending these studies in an attempt to provide further evidence for the importance of a genetic predisposition in determining the cardiovascular and physiological responses to environmental stress and dietary salt loading in man.

Within the kidney there are clearly many sites at which a genetic abnormality could predispose to sodium retention in the face of increasing delivery of sodium to the renal tubule and/or increasing renal sympathetic efferent nerve activity. A number of studies have recently suggested that genetic factors may determine the way in which renal proximal tubular cell surface receptors adapt to the influence of dietary salt loading. For example, in some salt sensitive strains of rats, renal tubular alpha-2 adrenoceptors increase in response to dietary salt intake in contrast to salt-resistant strains in which no such up-regulation of adrenoceptors occurs. These receptors, which it is believed are coupled negatively to adenylate cyclase, following alpha stimulation may facilitate the proximal tubular sodium hydrogen antiport system. This up-regulation of α-adrenoceptors could be a genetically determined mechanism facilitating sodium reabsorption in susceptible individuals [21]. Returning to the human model, we therefore propose that variations in the immediate response to migration might be explained by the interaction of the two environmental factors, stress and dietary sodium, which in genetically susceptible subjects leads to an increase in renal tubular sodium and water reabsorption and an initial volume dependent rise in blood pressure. The genetic abnormality proposed may also be represented in other tissues such as vascular smooth muscle cells where adrenoceptor linked stimulation of the sodium hydrogen antiporter will enhance vascular reactivity and increase vascular resistance.

In the present studies a high proportion of the migrants fail to "adapt" to migration, at least in terms of the blood pressure response, and this may well be a reflection of the ethnic group studied. In an evolutionary sense, in the arid climes of central Africa, the ability to conserve salt and water would constitute a biological advantage. However, the process of natural selection would favour conservers, but in the new (westernised) or urban environment where salt and water are both readily available, the advantage is reversed.

Further analyses are currently underway to look at the longer term blood pressure responses to the migration process. Of interest is the apparent relationship between the variables and systolic and diastolic pressure in the two sexes at different time points following migration and although the analyses are by no means complete, the data suggest that the factors that determine not only absolute levels of blood pressure, but also the relationship between blood pressure and age, vary with time. For example, the association between "neurogenic" factors as evidenced by pulse rate and blood pressure appear to become less important after the early 0–3 months following migration, for example. Other interesting observations concern preliminary findings on a subgroup of migrants who returned to their native villages. Blood pressure responses eventually reverse, but slowly, and in some, many months pass before blood pressure begins to fall. This would be compatible with the concept that structural changes develop in the vasculature of the urban migrants and these play an increasingly important part in determining levels of vascular resistance and hence blood pressure as time goes by, thereby reducing the impact of the neurogenic component. Such vascular changes would explain why blood pressure changes with reverse migration occur over a longer period of time than the acute changes occurring in the early stages of migration.

## Conclusion

These studies carried out in East Africa reveal a dramatic and rapid increase in blood pressure with migration from a subsistence farming rural environment to the urban slums of Nairobi. We suggest that this process represents a new dynamic model for essential hypertension in man.

The hypothesis proposed is that genetically determined failure of adaptation to the combined effects of environmental stress and an increase in dietary sodium explains the early change in blood pressure. By analogy with certain experimental models of hypertension in the rat, the locus of the underlying genetic abnormality could be in the central nervous system facilitating sympathetic outflow to the kidney in response to stress, or in the kidney facilitating sodium reabsorption when dietary salt is increased and renal sympathetic activity is maintained. The failure of homeostatic adjustment to the new environment, or failure of adaptation in a high proportion of migrants, suggests that sodium conserving mechanisms may have been highly developed in this ethnic group and that relatively free access to sodium in a stressful urban environment is an important determinant of the early blood pressure rise.

*Acknowledgement*

The data upon which this hypothesis was based could not have been provided without the help and assistance of a very large number of people. The authors would like to thank The Wellcome Trust for their extensive support for this research project. They would also like to express their gratitude to the people of the community served by the Saradidi Rural Health Project, and to Claire Poulter and Jan Lury for their commitment and help in obtaining most of the data on which the analyses were subsequently undertaken.

**References**

1. Poulter N, Khaw KT, Hopwood BEC, Mugambi M, Peart WS, Rose G, Sever PS (1984a) Blood pressure and its correlates in an African tribe in urban and rural environments. J Epid Comm Health 38:181–186
2. Poulter N, Khaw KT, Hopwood BEC, Mugambi M, Peart WS, Rose G, Sever PS (1984b) Blood pressure and associated factors in a rural Kenyan community. Hypertension 6:810–813
3. Poulter N, Khaw KT, Hopwood BEC, Mugambi M, Peart WS, Sever PS (1985) Determinants of blood pressure due to urbanisation – a longitudinal study. J Hypertension 3 (Suppl 3):375–377
4. Intersalt Co-operative Research Group (1988) Intersalt: an international study of electrolyte excretion and blood pressure. Results for 24 hour urinary sodium and potassium excretion. Br Med J 297:319–328
5. Pickering personal communication
6. Beaglehole R, Salmond CE, Hooper A, Huntsman J, Stanhope JM, Carsel JC, Prior IAM (1977) Blood pressure and social interaction in Tokelauan migrants in New Zealand. J Chron Dis 30:803–812
7. Dietz R, Schonig A, Haebara H, Mann JFE, Rascher W, Luth JB, Grunherz N, Gross F (1978) Studies on the pathogenesis of spontaneous hypertension of rats. Hypertension 43(Suppl):98–106
8. Koepke JP, di Bona GF (1985a) Central b-adrenergic receptors mediate renal nerve activity during stress in conscious SHR. Hypertension 7:350–356
9. Koepke JP, di Bona GF (1985b) High sodium intake enhances renal nerve and antinatriuretic responses to stress in spontaneously hypertensive rats. Hypertension 7:357–563
10. Dargie HJ, Franklin SS, Reid JL (1977) Plasma noradrenaline concentrations in experimental renovascular hypertension in the rat. Clin Sci Mol Med 52:477–483
11. Reid JL, Zivin JA, Kopin IJ (1975) Central and peripheral adrenergic mechanisms in the development of deoxycorticosterone-saline hypertension in rats. Circ Res 37:569–579
12. Koepke JP, Jones S, di Bona GF (1986) Renal nerve activity and renal function during environmental stress in DOCA-NaCl rats. Am J Physiol 251 (Regulatory Integrative Comp Physiol 20):R289–294
13. De Fronzo RA (1981) The effect of insulin on renal sodium metabolism. Diabetologia 21:165–171

14. Moden M, Halkin H, Almog S, Lusky A, Eshkol A, Shefi M, Shitrit A, Fuchs Z (1985) Hyperinsulinaemia: A link between hypertension, obesity and glucose intolerance. J Clin Invest 75:809–817

15. Scotch NA, Geiger JH (1963) Epidemiology of essential hypertension: psychologic and socio-cultural factors in etiology. J Chronic Dis 16:1183–1213

16. Cruz-Coke R, Etcheverry R, Nagel R (1964) Influence of migration on the blood pressure of Easter Islanders. Lancet I:697–699

17. Takeda K, Bunag RD (1980) Augmented sympathetic nerve activity and pressor responsiveness in DOCA hypertensive rats. Hypertension 2:97–101

18. Bianchi G, Fox U, Di Francesco GF, Giovannetti AM, Pagetti D (1974) Blood pressure changes produced by kidney cross-transplantation between spontaneously hypertensive rats and normotensive rats. Clin Sci Mol Med 47:435–448

19. Guidi E, Bianchi G, Rivolta E, Ponticelli C, Quarto di Palo F, Minetti L, Polli E (1985) Hypertension in man with a kidney transplant: role of familial versus other factors. Nephron 41:14–21

20. Light KC, Koepke JP, Obrist PA, Willis PW, IV (1983) Psychological stress induces sodium and fluid retention in men at high risk for hypertension. Science 220:429–431

21. Insel PA, Snavely MD, Healy DP, Munzel PA, Potenza CL, Nord EP (1985) Radioligand binding and functional assays demonstrate postsynaptic alpha$_2$-receptors on proximal tubules of rat and rabbit kidney. J Cardiovasc Pharmacol 7 (Suppl 8):9–17

Authors address:
Professor P. S. Sever
Department of Clinical Pharmacology,
St. Mary's Hospital Medical School,
London W2 1NY.
UK

# Neurogenic aspects of blood pressure control in man – with an emphasis on renovascular hypertension

C. J. Mathias, J. S. Kooner

Medical Unit, St Mary's Hospital and Medical School, London and University Department of Clinical Neurology, Institute of Neurology, National Hospital for Nervous Diseases, Queen Square, London, UK.

## Introduction

The earliest direct link between the nervous system and vascular control appears to have been made in 1727 by Pourfois du Petit [57] who observed dilatation of conjunctival vessels after section of the cervical sympathetic nerves in the rabbit. Considerable information has since been collected on how the nervous system influences blood pressure at a cerebral, spinal, and peripheral nerve level, in addition to its actions on the release of hormones with vaso-active properties, and its effects on organs which affect the circulation, such as the kidney. Advances have occurred despite the difficulties encountered in studying human subjects, especially in disorders such as hypertension where there may be multiple and variable effects on different organs. Some of the approaches which have broadened our concepts on neurogenic control of blood pressure are outlined (Table 1), and the application of some of these to patients with reno-vascular hypertension is described.

**Table 1.** Some of the approaches utilized in studying neural control of the circulation in man

| | |
|---|---|
| 1) Physiological | – Increasing sympathetic activity by "pressor tests" – cutaneous cold, isometric exercise<br>– Baroreceptor reflex assessment – physiological or pharmacological<br>– Microneuronography – measurement of skin and muscle sympathetic efferent activity |
| 2) Biochemical | – Plasma catecholamine measurements<br>– Measurement of catecholamine metabolites in cerebrospinal fluid, blood and urine<br>– Plasma dopamine beta hydroxylase measurements |
| 3) Pharmacological | – Ganglionic blockers – hexamethonium<br>– Alpha and beta adrenoceptor blockers<br>– Centrally acting agents – clonidine |
| 4) Patients with neurological disorders | – Spinal cord lesions – especially high cervical cord transection<br>– Chronic autonomic failure<br>– Peripheral lesions such as brachial plexus injuries<br>– Localized cerebral lesions – due to tumors, cerebrovascular accidents, congenital malformations |
| 5) Neuro-imaging | – Magnetic Resonance Imaging<br>– Positron Emission Tomography |

**Approaches to studying neurogenic control of the circulation in man**

*Physiological*

In the 1930s attempts to determine neurogenic dependence in hypertension was by the use of stimuli such as immersion of the hand in cold water and isometric exercise, which raised blood pressure reflexly through stimulation of sympathetic neural activity. Greater responses were observed in patients with hypertension [1, 18] but it was unclear if these resulted from exaggerated neural activity or enhanced cardiovascular reactivity. Understanding of the former emphasized the need to evaluate the different components of the baro-receptor reflex pathways, the major neural determinants of blood pressure control. In 1925, MacWilliam [26] noted that slowing of the pulse with elevation of blood pressure (Marey's reflex) was impaired in hypertensives. A variety of elegant approaches [19] have since extended our knowledge of circulatory reflexes in man and confirmed that baro-reflex sensitivity is abnormal in different groups of hypertensives. The specific site of the abnormality however remains difficult to determine, and there is uncertainty about whether it initiates, or results from, the hypertensive process. In specific situations this has been resolved by direct nerve recordings, as in patients after carotid endarterectomy where activity of the carotid sinus nerves is closely linked to changes in blood pressure [2]. The direct recording of muscle and skin efferent sympathetic activity in conscious man, using the microneurographic technique pioneered by Wallin [64] has extended our knowledge of sympathetic efferent nerve activity in a variety of situations in normotensive and hypertensive man, despite the limitation that measurements are made in a specific territory.

*Biochemical*

The early part of the 20th century was marked by numerous advances in understanding the chemical basis of autonomic activity. A key breakthrough in the 1940s was the recognition that noradrenaline, and not adrenaline, was the major neurotransmitter at sympathetic nerve endings [15]. This was confirmed by Peart [53] who, by parallel pharmacological assay, demonstrated noradrenaline release in venous blood on stimulating the sympathetic nerves of the cat spleen. Knowledge of the mechanisms accounting for the release, metabolism, and clearance of noradrenaline, together with refinements in sensitivity and specificity of its measurement have extended our understanding and utilization of plasma noradrenaline levels as an index of sympathetic neural activity in various physiological and pathological states [13, 16]. Other more controversial biochemical approaches include measurement of metabolites of catecholamines such as 3-methoxy 4-hydroxyphenylglycol (MHPG) in cerebrospinal fluid, which may indicate brain noradrenaline turnover [56]. The enzyme dopamine beta-hydroxylase converts dopamine into noradrenaline and is released stoichiometrically with the latter; plasma levels of this enzyme may have been a more useful marker of sympathetic activity as it is not influenced by uptake and metabolism, but the initial promise has unfortunately not been fulfilled [65].

*Pharmacological*

In the 1950s the first specifically targeted anti-hypertensive agents became available for use in man. Ganglionic blockers such as hexamethonium prevented post-ganglionic sympathetic and parasympathetic activity, and were highly successful in lowering blood pressure, although at the expense of several, sometimes serious side effects [52, 59]. It was hoped that they would help differentiate neurogenic from non-neurogenic factors in hypertension, and the greater fall in blood pressure induced by hexamethonium in patients with essential hypertension was provided as evidence of autonomic hyperactivity [12]. Advances in receptor pharmacology have led to drugs with selectivity and specificity for both pre- and post-synaptic receptors and thus the better definition of peripheral autonomic and vascular activity. In man there have however been few agents which act on the central nervous system to lower blood pressure. The most extensively studied is the alpha-2 adrenoceptor agonist, clonidine, which exerts its hypotensive effects predominantly by its central actions and has thus been a valuable neuropharmacological probe in dissecting dependence on neurogenic mechanisms [23, 31, 58] (Fig. 1).

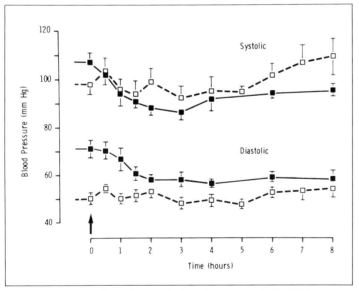

**Fig. 1a.** Mean systolic and diastolic blood pressures ($\pm$ SEM) in normal subjects (filled squares, continuous line) and in tetraplegic patients (open squares and interrupted lines) before and after 300 mcg of clonidine (indicated by an arrow). In the normal subjects there was a fall in both systolic and diastolic blood pressure, which remained low for eight h after drug administration. In the tetraplegics however, there was no fall in blood pressure. Clonidine caused a similar degree of sedation and dryness of mouth in both groups indicating similar central side effects. The plasma clonidine concentrations were also similar in the two groups. These studies therefore indicate that in man, integrity of descending sympathetic pathways is necessary for the hypotensive action of clonidine (from [58]).

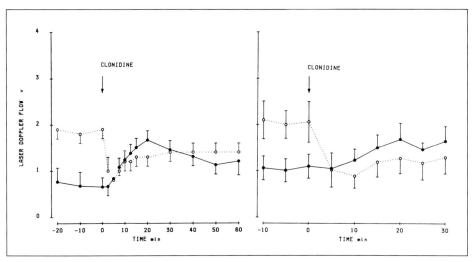

**Fig. 1 b.** Skin blood flow over the index finger measured by laser doppler flowmetry (in volts) before and after iv clonidine (given at time 0 as a 10 min infusion of 2 mcg/kg). The left panel indicates responses in normal subjects (filled circles, continuous lines) and tetraplegic patients (open circles and interrupted lines). In the normal subjects after clonidine there is digital cutaneous vasodilatation, which reaches its maximum after 20 min. In the tetraplegics the basal flow is higher, consistent with diminished sympathetic tone. After clonidine, however, there is a reduction in flow and calculation of resistance changes indicates vasoconstriction with some recovery over the period of observation. The right panel indicates responses to a similar dose of clonidine in patients with brachial plexus injuries, with simultaneous recordings in the innervated (filled circles, continuous line) and denervated (open circles and interrupted line) limbs. In the denervated limb there was a complete post-ganglionic sympathetic lesion. The responses in the innervated limb are similar to those in normal subjects, while those in the denervated limb are similar to those observed in the tetraplegics. In a vascular bed largely controlled by the central sympathetic nervous system this further emphasises that these responses to clonidine are abolished by either a pre- or a post-ganglionic sympathetic lesion.

*Study of patients with neurological lesions*

Since the 1960s there has been increasing awareness that the study of patients with neurological disorders can provide valuable information on neurogenic control of the circulation. Precise knowledge of the nature and site of the neurological lesion is of importance, as exemplified by the study of patients with complete cervical spinal cord transection, which is often the result of trauma. Tetraplegics are ideal physiological models of sympathetic decentralisation, as the brain is functionally separated from the spinal and peripheral sympathetic nervous systems; they therefore have postural hypotension because of their inability to reflexly activate sympathetic vasoconstrictor pathways, as would occur in normal subjects. These patients also exhibit "spinal autonomy", and reflex spinal sympathetic activity can occur as observed by Guttmann and Whitteridge [17] who recorded severe hypertension during stimulation of the urinary bladder. The paroxysmal hypertension is secondary to activation of cutaneo-, viscero- and somatovascular reflexes with afferents in skin, viscera, or muscle, increasing sympathetic efferent activity via the spinal cord [34]. Constriction in both resistance and capacitance vessels, a rise in cardiac output and an elevation in plasma noradrenaline but not plasma adrenaline levels is associated with the rise in blood pressure. In normal man these reflexes presumably activate cerebral mechanisms, among other factors, which mask the primary effect of such reflex stimulation and prevent the rise in blood pressure. The physiological, biochemical, and pharmacological investigations performed in these patients have defined the pathophysiological basis of some of their cardiovascular abnormalities, and additionally contributed to our understanding of the role of the sympathetic nervous system in hormonal and cardiovascular regulation [44]. These include studies on renin release mechanisms, especially in the absence of sympathetic activation [27, 32, 33], on the merits of plasma noradrenaline and plasma dopamine betahydroxylase as markers of sympathetic neural activity [29, 30], and on dissecting central from peripheral sites of action of drugs with multiple effects such as the competitive angiotensin-II antagonist saralasin [36, 63] and the alpha-2 adrenoceptor agonist clonidine [23, 31, 58] (see Figs. 1–4).

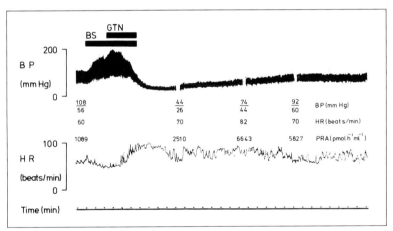

**Fig. 2a.** Rise in blood pressure (BP) during bladder stimulation (BS) induced by suprapubic percussion of the anterior abdominal wall in a chronic tetraplegic in the supine position. There is a rapid elevation in blood pressure, which may reach levels of > 200 mmHg systolic. There is usually a fall in heart rate, as a result of the vagal response to stimulation of intact baroreceptor afferents. Sublingual glyceryl trinitrate (GTN) (0.5 mgm for 3.5 min) rapidly reverses the hypertension elevates the heart rate (HR) and then causes substantial hypotension. This exaggerated depressor response reflects the inability to activate descending sympathetic efferent pathways in response to vasdilatation, as is observed in such patients during head-up tilt. The breaks in the record indicate where blood was withdrawn for measurement of plasma renin activity levels (PRA) which rise in response to the fall in blood pressure (from [44]).

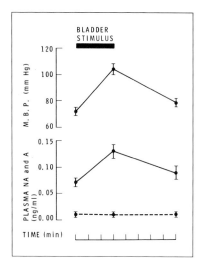

Fig. 2 b.

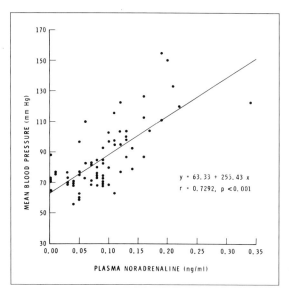

Fig. 2 c.

**Fig. 2 b, d, c and e.** 2 b and d indicate the changes in mean blood pressure (MBP) in a group of tetraplegic patients before, during, and after bladder stimulation. In 2 b are shown the changes in plasma noradrenaline (NA) and adrenaline (A) levels. The latter rise with the blood pressure and fall as the pressor effects wane. There is no change in plasma adrenaline levels. In 2 d levels of plasma dopamine beta hydroxylase rise slowly and remain elevated for a longer period. There is a strong relationship between blood pressure and plasma noradrenaline levels (2 c) which is not shown for plasma dopamine beta hydroxylase (2 e). Although dopamine beta-hydroxylase is released stoichiometrically with noradrenaline from the nerve terminal it presumably does not enter the circulation by the same route – it is a larger molecule and it probably utilizes alternative channels such as the lymphatics. In short-term studies in particular, plasma noradrenaline is a far better indicator of sympathetic neural activation, than plasma dopamine beta hydroxylase (from [28–30]).

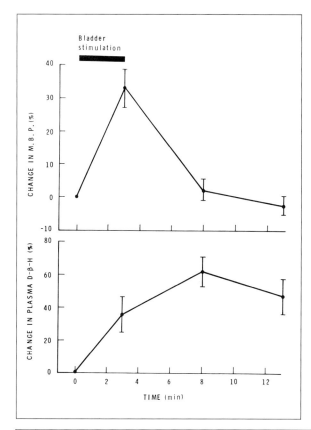

**Fig. 2 d.**

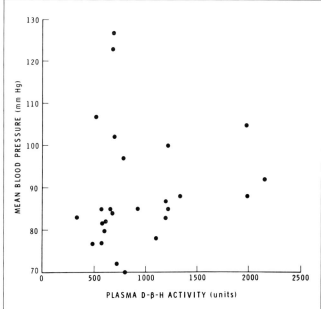

**Fig. 2 e.**

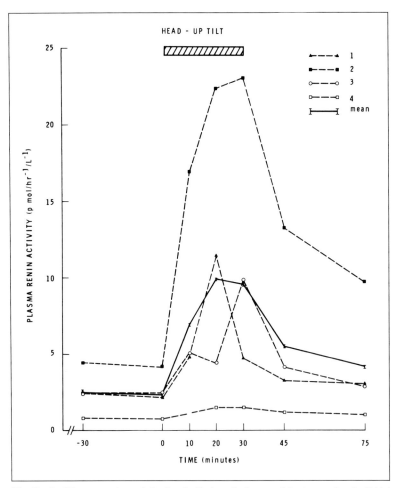

**Fig. 3a, b.** Plasma renin activity levels (3 a) and plasma aldosterone levels (3 b) in four tetraplegic patients while supine and horizontal ($-30$ and 0), 10, 20, and 30 min after 45° head-up tilt, and 45 and 75 min after the start of head-up tilt when they had returned to horizontal position for 15 and 45 min respectively. There was a prompt and substantial rise in levels of renin, except in patient 4 who had only a small fall in blood pressure during head-up tilt. There was little change in plasma noradrenaline levels during head-up tilt, indicating impairment of sympathetic vasoconstrictor activity. The rise in plasma aldosterone levels occurred later and was probably secondary to the elevation in renin and angiotensin-II levels, although impaired hepatic clearance may have contributed (from [27]).

**Fig. 3c.** Plasma renin activity levels in a group of tetraplegic patients before, during, and after head-up tilt to 45°. To exclude $\beta$-adrenoreceptor stimulation in the renin response to head-up tilt, patients were observed before and during $\beta$-adrenoreceptor blockade with iv propranolol. After propranolol there was no fall in basal levels of plasma renin activity. Head-up tilt resulted in a similar fall in blood pressure with no attenuation of the renin response to tilt (from [32]). These studies provide further evidence that renin release may occur independently of sympathetic and $\beta$-adrenoreceptor stimulation, and are probably dependent on activation of intrarenal baroreceptors following reduction in renal perfusion pressure.

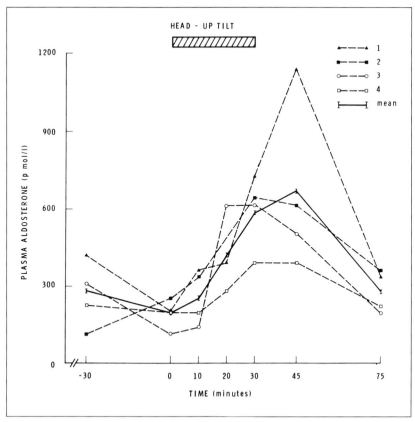

**Fig. 3 b.**

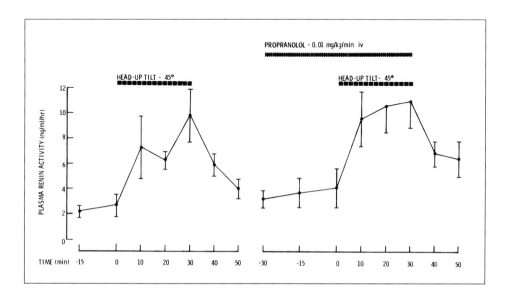

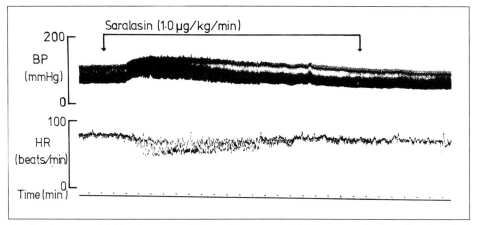

**Fig. 4a.** Intra-arterial blood pressure (BP) and heart rate (HR) in a tetraplegic patient in spinal shock before, during, and after intravenous infusion of saralasin (1 mcg m$^{-1}$ kg$^{-1}$). In spinal shock, which is present in the early stages after a spinal cord transection, there is a smaller likelihood of activating isolated spinal cord reflexes. Similar responses were also observed in a group of chronically-injured tetraplegic patients, suggesting that the transient pressor response to saralasin occurs independently of sympathetic nervous activity (from [36]).

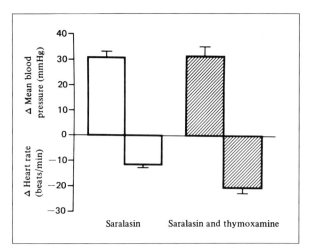

**Fig. 4b.** To further exclude stimulation of $\delta$-adrenoreceptors saralasin was infused before and after $\alpha$-adrenoreceptor blockade with thymoxamine. Histograms denote the maximum change ($\Delta$) in mean blood pressure and heart rate in the tetraplegic patients given 5 mcg of saralasin m$^{-1}$ kg$^{-1}$. There was a similar pressor response after thymoxamine, further emphasising that the pressor response caused by saralasin was independent of $\alpha$-adrenoreceptor stimulation and was likely to be an angiotensin-II-like agonist effect (from [36]).

Another group of patients who have enhanced our knowledge of neurogenic mechanisms in circulatory control are patients with chronic autonomic failure. They are a heterogenous group in whom the common feature is diffuse impairment of the sympathetic and often parasympathetic nervous systems; the cause is usually not known and the lesion may be central and/or peripheral [3]. The cardinal feature of this condition is postural hypotension, as they lack the ability to activate sympathetic vasoconstrictor nerves. Their hypotension is often more severe than in the tetraplegics, probably because of their inability to increase sympathetic activity at a spinal level and additionally because release of vasoactive hormones such as renin and vasopressin is often impaired. Investigation of such patients has provided valuable information on the role of the autonomic nervous system in a variety of clinically important situations [4]; these include the interactions between the kidney, hormones and salt and water homeostasis [22, 38, 66], and between food ingestion and release of pancreatic and gut peptides [37, 43]. The former can result in substantial nocturnal polyuria and worsening of morning postural hypotension [38] while the latter may cause severe postprandial hypotension (Fig. 5). Post-prandial hypotension appears largely related to carbohydrate and fat intake and to release of vaso-dilatatory peptides such as insulin and neurotensin [41, 43]. Haemodynamic studies indicate that food ingestion induces marked splanchnic vasodilatation, which is not accompanied in the patients by a compensatory rise in cardiac output and constriction in skeletal muscle vasculature, which depend on an intact sympathetic nervous system. Pretreatment with the somatostatin analogue SMS201-995 (octreotide) inhibits peptide release and effectively prevents post-prandial hypotension, further emphasising the role of peptides released during food ingestion [45]. These studies emphasise the importance of the splanchnic circulation in blood pressure control, which is reminiscent of the interest 50 years ago 51 when splanchnic denervation was used in the management of severe hypertension. A number of the peptides released during food ingestion are neuropeptides co-released with the major classical neurotransmitters at nerve endings [25] and have autonomic and vascular effects, which need further definition.

Systemic or regional cardiovascular abnormalities occur in a wide variety of neurological disorders [40] and their study is of importance in improving clinical management and understanding neural control mechanisms.

*Modern neuro-imaging*

Since the 1970s there have been several technical achievements which now enable more precise definition of the site and nature of neurological diseases, using non-invasive techniques. Nuclear magnetic resonance imaging, especially in combination with gadolinium, is of particular value in disorders affecting the brain stem, where lesions as small as 0.2 mm can be delineated [50] (Fig. 5). Positron emission tomography scanning using labelled amino-acid precursors and ligands provides in vivo knowledge of cerebral neurotransmitters and their sites of action [7] (Figs. 6, 7). With appropriate antagonists both pre- and postsynaptic receptors and their subtypes can be defined. This has been successfully applied to the central dopaminergic system and ligands for mapping central adrenoceptor subtypes are becoming in-

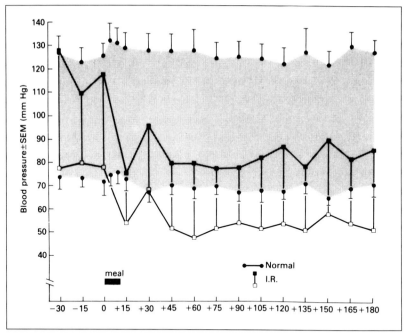

**Fig. 5a.** Supine systolic and diastolic blood pressure before and after a standard meal in a group of normal subjects (stippled area) ±SEM and in a patient with chronic autonomic failure (IR, continuous lines). Blood pressure does not change in the normal subjects, while in the patient there is a rapid fall to levels as low as 80/50 mmHg, which remain low even in the supine position over the three-h observation period. Food ingestion can thus considerably enhance postural hypotension (from [43]) (Fig. 5 b). Percentage changes in mean blood pressure in 6 patients with autonomic failure given either a standard meal, or an isocaloric and isovolemic solution of carbohydrate (glucose, 1 g/kg body weight), lipid (Prosperol 0.95 ml/kg) or protein (Maxipro 1 g/kg) alone. Vertical bars indicate ±SEM (from [43]). The changes after glucose mimic the responses after a meal.

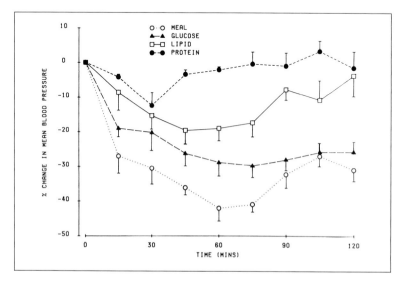

**Fig. 5 b.**

creasingly available. These advances in neuro-imaging should enable even greater precision in the ability to correlate neurological disorders with neurotransmitter and associated cardiovascular deficits, and thus provide the basis for reversal of abnormalities with appropriate pharmacological agents.

## The future

It is clear from the brief descriptions above that we are now in an exciting position in our endeavours to discover more about the neurogenic control of the circulation in man. We have knowledge of the basic processes involved in neurotransmission, availability of sensitive biochemical assays, accessibility of non-invasive methods to study neural and cardiovascular function and useful leads from patients with neurological disorders. This should further help in determining the role of the nervous system in a wide range of cardiovascular disorders and will hopefully determine if neurogenic influences contribute to the elevation in blood pressure in the large group of patients with "essential hypertension", in whom many initiating factors have been postulated but where few of the theories have been substantiated.

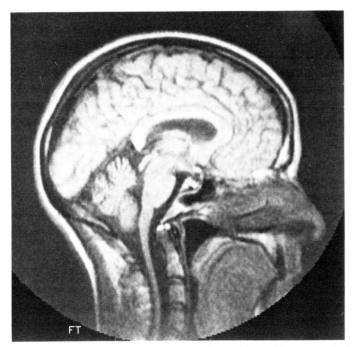

**Fig. 6.** Magnetic resonance imaging scan in a patient with autonomic dysfunction, cardiovascular abnormalities, cerebellar and brain stem deficits. This section shows loss of the normal flocculation in parts of the cerebellum. There also appear to be brain stem defects.

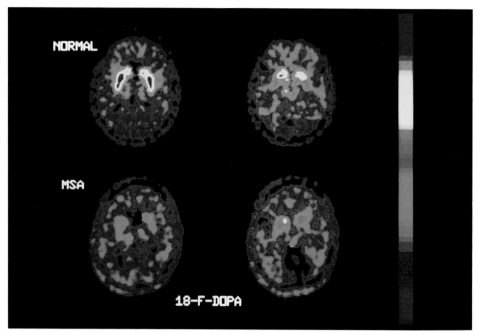

**Fig. 7.** Positron emission tomography scan in a normal subject and in a patient with multiple system atrophy (MSA) and chronic autonomic failure. This patient also had extrapyramidal symptoms and signs. Scanning following 18-f-dopa administration indicates that its conversion into dopamine is impaired in the patient with MSA. The normal distribution within the basal ganglia (shown in yellow and red) in the head of the caudate and the putamen is reduced in equivalent sections from the MSA patient (from [7]).

## Neurogenic mechanisms in human renovascular hypertension

It is commonly accepted that hypertension in patients with renal artery stenosis is secondary to activation of the renin-angiotensin system and elevated angiotensin-II (AII) levels. This concept was questioned 25 years ago by McCubbin and Page [46], who in dogs noted a greater elevation in blood pressure when sympathetic stimulation was induced by drugs (tyramine, ephedrine, or ganglionic stimulants), or activation of pressor reflexes (carotid occlusion) during infusion of sub-pressor doses of A-II. Recognition and localisation of the cerebral effects of A-II at sites such as the area postrema in the brainstem, together with identification of central A-II receptors [11, 20, 47] provided further insight into the mechanism by which humoro-neural coupling and activation of the nervous system may occur in renovascular hypertension. In patients with unequivocal renal artery stenosis, levels of renin/A-II may not be elevated and antagonism or inhibition of A-II does not

**Table 2.** Outline of the three phases of experimental 1 clip-2 kidney Goldblatt hypertension showing the relationship between blood pressure (BP), renin/A-II (angiotensin-II) levels, A-II antagonism by saralasin, A-II inhibition by captopril, and clip removal (revascularization) or nephrectomy

|  | Blood pressure | Renin/A-II levels | A-II antagonism or inhibition | Revascularization or nephrectomy |
|---|---|---|---|---|
| Phase I | Elevated | Elevated | BP reduced | BP reduced |
| Phase II | Elevated | Elevated or normal | BP unchanged or falls if drug-administration is prolonged | BP reduced |
| Phase III | Elevated | Normal or decreased | BP unchanged | BP unchanged |

necessarily lower blood pressure; in such patients the direct vascular effects of A-II seem unlikely to maintain hypertension and we have considered the possibility that alternative mechanisms, including those exerted through the nervous system, are responsible. We describe studies in patients with unilateral renal artery stenosis as their hypertension is more likely to be dependent on the effects of renal ischaemia than patients with bilateral stenosis, where renal impairment and subsequent salt and water retention are likely to play an important, if not dominant role.

*Phases in experimental renovascular hypertension*

In man the precise duration of the renal stenotic lesion and hypertension is difficult, if not impossible to determine. Longitudinal studies in equivalent animal models induced by a clip over one renal artery, with the contralateral renal vasculature and kidney intact (1 clip-2 kidney Goldblatt model) have provided information which may be relevant to human renovascular hypertension. There appear to be three reasonably distinct phases in such experimental models [8] (Table 2). Following renal artery clipping the blood pressure rises promptly, with an elevation of renin/A-II levels (Phase I); the hypertension is abolished by acute antagonism of A-II or inhibition of A-II production. Following this, blood pressure remains elevated while levels of renin/A-II fall (Phase II). Acute antagonism of A-II or inhibition of A-II formation usually does not lower blood pressure unless administration of these agents is prolonged. In Phase II, as in Phase I, the ischaemic kidney is responsible for the hypertension as revascularisation (by clip removal) or nephrectomy restores the blood pressure to previous levels. This suggests that in Phase II mechanisms working independently of, or in addition to, the direct vascular effects of A-II are involved. This phase is followed by the irreversible phase of hypertension, Phase III, when blood pressure does not fall, despite the use of drugs, revascularisation or nephrectomy; changes such as hypertrophy of blood vessels and heart and/or damage to the contralateral kidney have probably occurred and may maintain the hypertension.

These experimental observations may be important in the human situation. In our experience it is likely that the majority of our patients fall into the reversible phases of hypertension, which can be ameliorated or cured by revascularization or removal of the ischaemic kidney [14]. Whether these patients fall into Phase I or II needs to be defined by their levels of renin/A-II and blood pressure responses to A-II antagonism or inhibition. Patients with normal or modestly elevated levels of renin/ A-II and with minimal depressor responses to the latter drug, probably fall into the experimental Phase II. In this phase the mechanisms accounting for the hypertension are debated even in animals, as there is a clear dissociation between the elevated blood pressure and renin levels. A "slow pressor component" of A-II has been postulated with sodium retention as a causative factor [9]. This has not been supported experimentally [62] and an unfavourable redistribution of sodium, rather than its actual retention, has been subsequently argued for. We have hypothesized that in patients with clearly defined unilateral renal artery stenosis the nervous system plays an increasing and sometimes major role in the maintenance of hypertension and that this may be the missing or additional factor [39, 42].

*Assessing neurogenic mechanisms in human renovascular hypertension*

Our approach to determining neural control was to study the haemodynamic and hormonal effects of the neuropharmacological probe, clonidine in patients with clearly defined ulilateral renal artery stenosis. In the same patients the dependency of the hypertension on the peripheral effects of circulating A-II was determined by comparing the responses after the A-I converting enzyme inhibitor captopril. A total of 33 patients with unilateral renal artery stenosis were studied. All underwent flush aortography and selective renal angiography to confirm the diagnosis. In the majority, investigations included intravenous urography, isotope renography, and divided renal vein renin measurements; in some the initial diagnosis was made on intravenous digital subtraction angiography [14]. Hypertension was severe in the majority and had often been difficult to control even on a combination of three or more drugs, which included diuretics, beta adrenoceptor blockers and vasodilators. The cause of the stenosis was atheroma in the majority and fibromuscular hyperplasia in the rest. Follow up in our patients indicated that hypertension in the majority was ameliorated or cured by interventional procedures such as angioplasty, revascularization surgery, or nephrectomy, indicating that the stenosis was not coincidental and either caused or contributed to the hypertension.

Patients were studied after they had been off antihypertensive medication for at least three days. Non-invasive measurements were made; using an automated sphygmomanometer for blood pressure and heart rate, mercury in silastic strain gauge plethysmography for forearm bloodflow, multiple thermistors as an index of cutaneous bloodflow, laser Doppler flowmetry to assess changes in the capillary bed of the index finger and a continuous wave Doppler technique for cardiac output. From a venous cannula blood was collected for measurements of plasma renin activity and plasma aldosterone (by radio-immunoassay) and plasma noradrenaline and adrenaline (radioenzymatic assay and high pressure liquid chromatography techniques).

*Haemodynamic and neuro-hormonal effects of clonidine*

The initial studies were performed with oral clonidine (300 µgm) which substantially lowered both systolic and diastolic blood pressure, the greatest fall being between two to four after administration [35] (Fig. 8 a). The low levels of blood pressure persisted for eight h, when observation stopped. There was a small fall in heart rate. There was no reduction in levels of plasma renin activity but plasma noradrenaline fell significantly (Fig. 8 b). This suggested that clonidine suppressed central pressor mechanisms, probably sympathetically mediated, to reduce blood pressure. Clonidine however has multiple effects, some independent of its central sympatholytic actions, which may alternatively have been responsible for the fall in blood pressure (Table 3). A series of studies was therefore performed to assess these possibilities.

**Table 3.** Some of the mechanisms, (independent of a reduction in sympathetic activity) by which clonidine may have lowered blood pressure in patients with renal artery stenosis

1. Suppression of renin release
2. Reduction of aldosterone secretion
3. Inhibition of vasopressin secretion
4. Diminution of intravascular volume
5. Antagonism of the pressor effects of angiotension – II

A group of patients was studied with intravenous clonidine, given in a dose of 2 µgm/kg over 10 min to avoid the initial transient pressor response which may occur because of its partial alpha-adrenergic agonist actions. Blood pressure fell substantially and remained low over an observation period of two h, with no reduction in levels of renin or aldosterone, confirming that suppression of the renin-angiotensin-aldosterone system did not contribute to the hypotension. Blood pressure remained low even when patients had recovered from the initial sedation and were essentially awake and alert. A group of patients, some with essential hypertension, were restudied after the benzodiazepine, nitrazepam, 10 mg orally, which caused a similar degree of sedation as confirmed on clinical observation and with visual analogue scales. There was however no fall in either blood pressure or plasma noradrenaline levels, making it unlikely that the substantial and prolonged hypotension after clonidine was secondary to its sedative effects.

In some experimental models arginine vasopressin may contribute to the maintenance of renovascular hypertension [48]. Plasma vasopressin levels were therefore measured (by Drs. Stafford Lightman and Meurig Williams) before and after clonidine. Basal levels of vasopressin were within the normal range and there was no fall after clonidine, indicating that the hypotension was independent of vasopressin inhibition. In animals the sympathetic nervous system has been shown to influence sodium and water homeostasis, and thus plasma volume, by actions on the gastrointestinal tract and renal tubules [60, 61]. Plasma osmolality, plasma electrolytes, and the haematrocrit were however unchanged after clonidine, making it unlikely that a reduction in intravascular volume contributed. A group of patients was

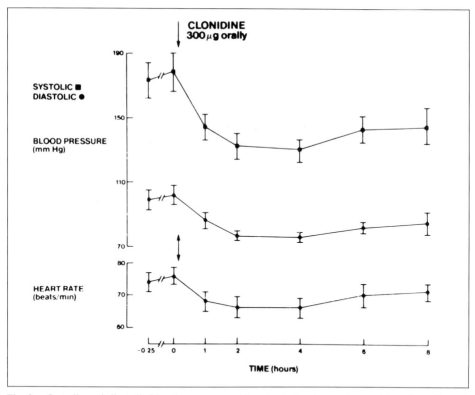

**Fig. 8 a.** Systolic and diastolic blood pressure and heart rate in nine patients with unilateral renal artery stenosis, before (−0.25 and 0) and one, two, four, six and eight h after 300 mcg of oral clonidine. There was a substantial fall in blood pressure which is maximal between the second and fourth hour and persisted until the end of the period of observation, eight h after administration of clonidine (Fig. 8 b). Plasma renin activity and plasma noradrenaline levels in the nine patients with unilateral renal artery stenosis at the same time points after oral clonidine. There is no change in levels of plasma renin during the study but there was a significant fall in plasma noradrenaline levels (from [35]).

studied after 20 mg of frusemide intravenously, which caused a marked diuresis but did not lower blood pressure, further excluding plasma volume depletion as a mechanism for the hypotensive effects of clonidine.

Low doses of clonidine over a prolonged period may antagonize the effect of vasopressor agents and this may account for its benefit in patients with migrainous headaches [67]. We therefore determined the pressor dose response curves to incremental intravenous infusions of A-II in a group of patients before and after clonidine. There was no reduction in the pressor response to A-II after clonidine, thus excluding peripheral antagonism of the vascular effects of A-II as a reason for the fall in blood pressure.

Our studies therefore indicate that the substantial and prolonged hypotensive effects of clonidine in patients with unilateral renal artery stenosis probably result from its central sympatholytic effects. These actions are consistent with results from

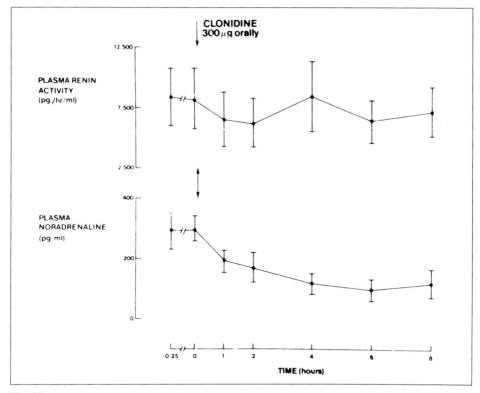

**Fig. 8b.**

detailed hemodynamic studies in such patients [24]. After clonidine there was a fall in cardiac output, with no change in skeletal muscle blood flow and in cutaneous blood flow except in the hand, which from previous studies [55], is known to be largely dependent on sympathetic vasoconstrictor nerve activity. This is in accord with the fall in plasma noradrenaline levels, which indicate an overall decrease in sympathetic nervous activity. It is likely that vasodilatation also occurred in other vascular territories, such as the large splanchnic bed, and that this contributed to the hypotensive actions of clonidine.

*Effects of antagonism or inhibition of formation of angiotensin-II*

To determine the direct effects of A-II in maintaining blood pressure the competitive A-II antagonist saralasin was infused intravenously into six patients. In the majority there was no fall in blood pressure, while all six had a depressor response after clonidine. Subsequent studies were conducted with the A-I converting enzyme inhibitor captopril, in a dose of 50 mg orally, which adequately prevents A-II formation. Captopril had variable hypotensive effects, which were closely related to the basal level of plasma renin activity (Fig. 9) the greatest individual fall occurring in a

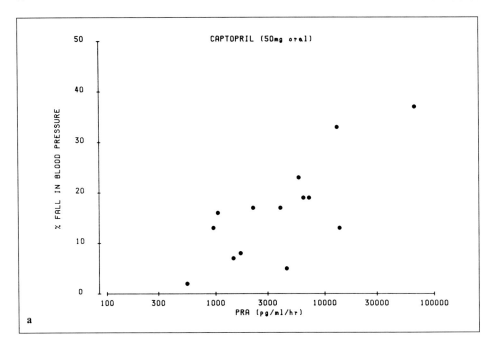

a

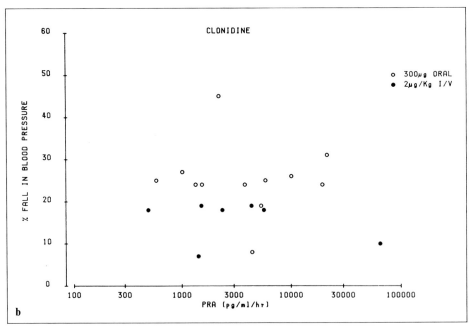

b

**Fig. 9 a, b.** Maximal hypotensive responses (percentage changes) to captopril (upper panel, 9 a) and clonidine (lower panel, 9 b) in 14 and 19 patients with unilateral renal artery stenosis, respectively. The blood pressure responses are plotted against basal plasma renin activity levels. There is a direct relationship between captopril induced hypotension and renin levels (r = 0.77, p < 0.01). The hypotension induced by clonidine bears no relationship to renin levels (from [39]).

patient with the highest circulating levels of renin (Fig. 10). In this patient clonidine had minimal hypotensive effects.

Detailed haemodynamic investigations indicated that after captopril there was a fall in cardiac output, which was similar to that observed after clonidine, but with little change in blood pressure, indicating that the hypotensive effects of clonidine were unlikely to be dependent on a decrease in cardiac output alone [24]. After captopril there were no changes in blood flow in either the cutaneous or skeletal muscle vasculature, and vasodilatation did not occur in the hand, as distinct from the effects observed after clonidine. After captopril, plasma noradrenaline levels did not fall, further indicating its inability to reduce sympathetic tone.

*What maintains hypertension in patients with unilateral renal artery stenosis?*

Our series of studies in patients with unilateral renal artery stenosis indicates that at least two major systems contribute to their hypertension. In the early stages, as in the experimental models, the renin-angiotensin symptom appears primarily responsible for initiating the hypertension. One of our patients had grossly elevated levels of renin and her blood pressure fell substantially after A-II inhibition with captopril but with little change after clonidine (Fig. 10). She had been followed closely over a long period and her clinical course and subsequent investigations indicated that she developed a critical renal artery stenosis only a few weeks prior to our studies. It is likely that she fell into Phase I of experimental 1 clip-2 kidney Goldblatt hypertension, and that the direct vascular effects of A-II initiated and maintained her hypertension.

The majority of our patients, however, had only a small fall in blood pressure after captopril, suggesting a lesser degree of dependence on the peripheral effects of A-II

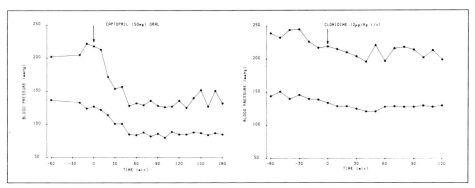

**Fig. 10.** Levels of systolic and diastolic blood pressure in a patient with extremely high levels of plasma renin activity (over 100,000 pcg/h/ml, normal range 500–15,000 pcg/h/ml) when given either captopril (left panel) or clonidine (right panel). After captopril there is a profound and sustained fall in blood pressure. Minimal changes only were observed after clonidine. The history, follow up and additional investigations in this patient indicated the recent development of a critical unilateral renal artery stenosis. She therefore appeared to fall into Phase I of experimental 1 clip – 2 kidney Goldblatt hypertension, which is largely dependent on the peripheral vascular effects of angiotensin-II.

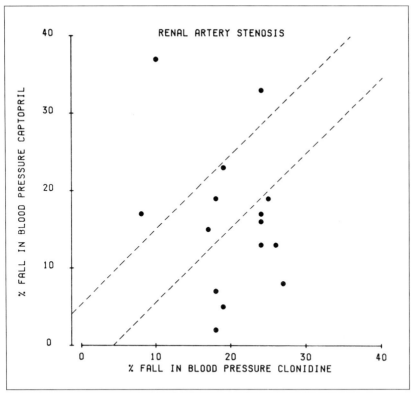

**Fig. 11.** Maximal (percentage) fall in blood pressure induced by clonidine plotted against maximum fall induced by captopril in 15 patients with unilateral renal artery stenosis. Patients whose responses fall within the stippled line are those in whom similar hypotensive responses were caused by either drug. Those to the left have had a considerably greater hypotensive response to captopril, indicating dependency on the peripheral circulating effects of angiotensin-II, while those on the right indicate a greater response to clonidine, suggesting that in them blood pressure was maintained by neurogenic mechanisms (from [39]).

(Fig. 11). These patients often had modestly elevated or normal renin levels and probably belonged to the later, Phase II of experimental renovascular hypertension where there is dissociation between renin levels and the hypertension. The "slow pressor component" of A-II or the "missing factor" responsible for maintaining hypertension in this phase is likely to involve the nervous system, as based on our observations with clonidine and on recent animal studies. Lesions of specific areas within the brain, such as the AV 3V region in the hypothalamus can prevent or reduce hypertension in animal models of renovascular hypertension [6]. The reason why such centres are activated in renovascular hypertension is unclear, but the cerebral actions of A-II, including those known to increase sympathetic nervous activity at other sites [68] may contribute. It may also be that increased sensitivity to A-II in the later phases of renovascular hypertension maintain such effects, despite a reduction in circulating A-II levels. Increased neurogenic activity may also result from stimulation of afferent renal nerves, and in experimental models peripheral denervation or interruption of their afferent pathways into the spinal cord by rhizotomy can prevent or reduce renovascular hypertension [21, 49]. Afferent renal nerves may be activated by either renal ischaemia or disease, which may explain why reduction of ischaemia by revascularization (angioplasty or surgery) or by nephrectomy, is effective in reducing hypertension in patients with renal artery stenosis.

*Implication of these studies*

These studies have reinforced the need to reconsider our concepts of the additional mechanisms which maintain an elevated blood pressure in patients with clearly defined secondary hypertension. The primary or initiating factor may in due course be superceded by factors such as activation of neurogenic mechanisms as we have demonstrated, or other factors including cardiac and vascular hypertrophy or renal damage. This may explain earlier observations by Peart [54] that definite removal of the primary cause of hypertension, such as the tumour in phaeochromocytoma patients, prevents hypertensive spikes but does not necessarily reduce persistent hypertension.

The role of multiple factors in blood pressure maintenance also emphasizes the need to consider the drawbacks of using the response to a specific pharmacological agent as a means of determining either the primary cause of hypertension or predicting the response to intervention. In our experience the hypotensive response to A-II inhibition with captopril was modest or minimal in a large number of patients with functional renal artery stenosis, whose hypertension was subsequently reduced or cured by revascularization procedures or nephrectomy. Its use as a predictor of response to intervention is therefore not recommended, especially when used acutely. When used on a long term basis in such patients it may reduce blood pressure, but the risk of potentially dangerous side effects which include the reduction of glomerular filtration and renal artery thrombosis may result in further irretrievable damage to an already ischaemic kidney. Awareness of additional mechanisms which maintain hypertension, such as those exerted through the nervous system, widens the choice of alternative antihypertensive agents which could be of value especially if long term therapy is needed in those patients in whom intervention is either not possible, is unsatisfactory, or has failed.

**Acknowledgements**

This review is a tribute to Professor Sir Stanley Peart, who has played a pivotal role in investigation of the neurogenic control of the circulation and has provided much inspiration, in addition to being an active participant in many of the studies described. CJM thanks his co-workers from the Churchill Hospital at Oxford, the National Spinal Injuries Centre at Stoke Mandeville Hospital, the Institute of Neurology and National Hospital for Nervous Diseases at Queen Square and St Mary's Hospital for their collaboration and help over the years. We particularly wish to thank two colleagues among many who have played a vital role – Sir Roger Bannister and Dr Hans Frankel, who enabled the study of patients with autonomic failure and spinal cord injury. CJM thanks the Wellcome Trust for their sustained support.

# References

1. Alam M, Smirk FH (1938) Blood pressure raising reflexes in health, essential hypertension and renal hypertension. Clin Sci 3:259–266

2. Angell-James JE, Lumley JSP (1971) The effects of carotid endarterectomy on the mechanical properties of the carotid sinus and carotid sinus nerves activity in atherosclerotic patients. Br J Surg 61:805–810

3. Bannister R (1988) Clinical features of autonomic failure. A. Symptoms, signs and special investigations. In: Bannister R (ed) Autonomic Failure: a textbook of clinical disorders of the autonomic nervous system. Second Edition. Oxford University Press, Oxford, pp 267–280

4. Bannister R, Mathias CJ (1988) Testing autonomic reflexes. In: Bannister R (ed) Autonomic Failure: a textbook of clinical disorders of the autonomic nervous system. Second Edition. Oxford University Press, Oxford pp 289–307

5. Birch R, Kooner JS, Mathias CJ, Peart WS, Stone F (1987) Clonidine induces differential changes in innervated and denervated limbs of humans with unilateral brachial plexus injury. J Physiol (London) 394:76 p.

6. Brody MJ, Johnson AK (1980) Role of the anteroventral third ventricle region in fluid and electrolyte balance, arterial pressure regulation and hypertension. In: Martini L, Ganong WF (eds) Frontiers in Neuroendocrinology. Raven Press, New York Vol 6:249–292

7. Brooks D, Salmon EP, Bannister R, Mathias CJ, Frackowiack R (1988) The integrity of the dopaminergic system in multiple system atrophy and pure autonomic failure studied with positron emission tomography. In: Proceedings of a Symposium on Movement Disorders, Manchester (in press)

8. Brown JJ, Cuesta V, Davies DL, Lever AF, Morton JJ, Padfield PL, Robertson JIS, Trust P, Bianchi G, Schalekamp MAD (1976) Mechanism of renal hypertension. Lancet I:1219–1221

9. Brown JJ, Lever AF, Robertson JIS (1979) Renal hypertension – aetiology, diagnosis and treatment. In: Black, Sir Douglas, Jones NF (eds) Renal disease, 4th edition, Blackwell Scientific Publications, Oxford 731–765

10. da Costa DF, Fosbraey P, Miller D, McDonald WI, Rudge P, Bannister R and Mathias CJ (1988) Abnormal cardiovascular autonomic reflexes and nuclear magnetic resonance scanning defects in patients with multiple sclerosis. J Neurol 235(Suppl):584

11. Dickenson CJ, Ferrario CM (1974) Central neurogenic effects of angiotensin. In: Page IH, Bumpus FM (eds) Angiotensin, Springer Berlin Heidelberg New York pp 408–416

12. Doyle AE, Smirk FH (1955) The neurogenic component in hypertension. Circulation 12:543–552

13. Esler MD, Hasking GJ, Willett IR, Lennard PW, Jennings GL (1985) Noradrenaline release and sympathetic nervous system activity. J Hypertension 3:117–129

14. Carmichael DJS, Mathias CJ, Snell ME, Peart WS (1986) Detection and investigation of renal artery disease. Lancet I:667–670

15. von Euler US (1946) Noradrenaline. CC Thomas, Springfield, Illinois

16. Goldstein DS, McCarty R, Polinsky RJ, Kopin IJ (1983) Relationship between plasma norepinephrine and sympathetic neural activity. Hypertension 5:552–559

17. Guttmann L, Whitteridge D (1947) Effects of bladder distension on autonomic mechanisms after spinal cord injury. Brain 70:361–404

18. Hines EA Jnr, Brown GE (1932) A standard stimulus for measuring vasomotor reactions: Its application in study of hypertension. Proc Mayo Clin 7:332–335

19. Jones JV, Sleight P (1981) Reflex control of the circulation in hypertensive humans. In: Abboud FM, Fozzard HA, Golmore JP, Reis DJ (eds) Disturbances in Neurogenic Control of the Circulation, American Physiological Society, Bethesda, pp 161–175

20. Joy MD, Lowe RD (1970) Evidence that the area postrema mediates the central cardiovascular response to angiotensin-II. Nature 228:1303–1304

21. Katholi RE, Whitlow PL, Winternitz SR, Oparil S (1982) Importance of the renal nerves in established two kidney, one clip Goldblatt hypertension. Hypertension 4(Suppl II):166–174

22. Kooner JS, da Costa DF, Frankel HL, Bannister R, Peart WS, Mathias CJ (1987) Recumbency induces hypertension, diuresis and natriuresis in autonomic failure but diuresis alone in tetraplegia. J Hypertension 5 (Suppl 5):327–329

23. Kooner JS, Edge W, Frankel HL, Peart WS, Mathias CJ (1988) Haemodynamic action of clonidine in tetraplegia – effects at rest and during bladder stimulation. Paraplegia 26:200–203

24. Kooner JS, Peart WS, Mathias CJ (1988) Cardiovascular and neurohormonal changes following central sympathetic blockade with clonidine in human unilateral renal artery stenosis. J Hypertension (in Press)

25. Lundberg JM, Hokfelt (1985) Co-existence of peptides and classical neurotransmitters. In: Bousfield D (ed) Neurotransmitters in Action, Elsevier Biomedical Press, Amsterdam, pp 104–118

26. MacWilliam JA (1925) Blood pressure in man under normal and pathological conditions. Physiol Rev 5:303

27. Mathias CJ, Christensen NJ, Corbett JL, Frankel HL, Goodwin TJ and Peart WS (1975) Plasma catecholamines, plasma renin activity and plasma aldosterone in tetraplegic man, horizontal and tilted. Clin Sci Mol Med 49:292–299

28. Mathias CJ (1976) Neurological Disturbances of the Cardiovascular System. Doctor of Philosophy Thesis, University of Oxford

29. Mathias CJ, Christensen NJ, Corbett JL, Frankel HL, Spalding JMK (1976) Plasma catecholamines during paroxysmal neurogenic hypertension in quadriplegic man. Circ Res 39:204–208

30. Mathias CJ, Smith AD, Frankel HL, Spalding JMK (1976) Release of dopamine B-hydroxylase during hypertension from sympathetic overactivity in man. Cardiovascular Res 10:176–181

31. Mathias CJ, Reid JL, Wing LMH, Frankel HL, Christensen NJ (1979) Antihypertensive effects of clonidine in tetraplegic subjects devoid of central sympathetic control. Clin Sci 57:425–428

32. Mathias CJ, Christensen NJ, Frankel HL, Peart WS (1980) Renin release during head-up tilt occurs independently of sympathetic nervous activity in tetraplegic man. Clin Sci 59:251–256

33. Mathias CJ, Frankel HL, Davies IB, James VHT, Peart WS (1981) Renin and aldosterone release during sympathetic stimulation in tetraplegia. Clin Sci 60:399–604

34. Mathias CJ, Frankel HL (1983) Autonomic failure in tetraplegia. In: Bannister R ed, Autonomic Failure: a textbook of clinical disorders of the autonomic nervous system, Oxford University Press, Oxford 453–488

35. Mathias CJ, Wilkinson AH, Lewis PL, Sever PS, Snell ME, Peart WS (1983) Clonidine lowers blood pressure independently of renin suppression in patients with unilateral renal artery stenosis. Chest 83:357–359

36. Mathias CJ, Unwin RJ, Pike FA, Frankel HL, Sever PS, Peart WS (1984) The immediate pressor response to saralasin in man: evidence against sympathetic activation and for intrinsic angiotensin-II-like myotropism. Clin Sci 66:517–524

37. Mathias CJ, da Costa DF, Fosbraey P, Bannister R, Christensen NJ (1986) Post-cibal hypotension in autonomic failure. In: Christensen NJ, Henricksen O, Lassen NA (eds) The Sympatho-adrenal System, Alfred Benzon Symposium No 23. Munksgaard, Copenhagen, pp 402–413

38. Mathias CJ, Fosbraey P, da Costa D, Thornley A, Bannister R (1986) Desmopressin reduces nocturnal polyuria, reverses overnight weight loss and improves morning postural hypotension in autonomic failure. Br Med J 293:353–354

39. Mathias CJ, Kooner JS, Peart WS (1986) Do neurogenic mechanisms maintain hypertension in renal artery stenosis? In: Gloriosa N, Laragh JH, Rappelli A (eds) Renovascular Hypertension: Pathophysiology, Diagnosis and Treatment. Raven Press, New York, pp 173–185

40. Mathias CJ (1987) Role of the central nervous system in human secondary hypertension. J Cardiovasc Pharmac 10 Suppl 12:93–99

41. Mathias CJ, da Costa DF, Fosbraey P, Christensen NJ, Bannister R (1987) Hypotensive and sedative effects of insulin in autonomic failure. Br Med J 295:161–163

42. Mathias CJ, Kooner JS, Peart WS (1987) Neurogenic components of hypertension in human renal artery stenosis. Clin Exp Hypertension A9(Suppl I):293–306

43. Mathias CJ, da Costa DF, Bannister R (1988) Post-cibal hypotension in autonomic disorders. In: Bannister R (ed) Autonomic Failure. A textbook of clinical disorders of the autonomic nervous system. Second edition. Oxford University Press, Oxford, pp 367–380

44. Mathias CJ, Frankel HL (1988) Cardiovascular control in spinal man. Ann Rev Physiol 50:577–592

45. Mathias CJ, Raimbach SJ, Cortelli T, Kooner JS, Bannister R (1988) The somatostatin analogue SMS 201-995 inhibits peptide release and prevents glucose-induced hypotension in autonomic failure. J Neurol 235(Suppl S):74–75

46. McCubbin JW, Page IH (1963) Neurogenic component of chronic renal hypertension. Science 139:210–211

47. Mendelsohn FAO, Quirion R, Saavedra JM, Aguilera G, Catt KJ (1984) Autoradiographic localization of angiotensin-II receptors in rat brain. Proc Natl Acad Sci USA 81:1575–1579

48. Mohring J (1978) Neurohypophyseal vasopressor principle: vasopressor hormone as well as antidiuretic hormone? Klin Wochenschr 56(Suppl):71–80

49. Oparil S, Wyss JM (1986) Neural-renal interactions: Evidence in experimental hypertension. In: Gloriosa N, Laragh JH, Rappelli A (eds) Renovascular Hypertension. Pathophysiology, diagnosis and treatment. Raven Press, New York, pp 125–158

50. Ormerod IEC, Miller DH, McDonald WI, du Boulay EPGH, Rudge P, Kendall BE, Moseley IF, Johnson G, Tofts PS, Halliday AM, Bronstein ALM, Scaravilli F, Harding AE, Barnes D, Zilkha KJ (1987) The role of NMR imaging in the assessment of multiple sclerosis and isolated neurological lesions. Brain 110:1579–1616

51. Page IH, Heuer GJ (1937) Effect of splanchnic nerve resection on patients suffering from hypertension. Am J Med Soc 193:820–841

52. Paton WDM, Zaimis EJ (1952) The methonium compounds. Pharmacol Rev 4:219–253

53. Peart WS (1949) The nature of splenic sympathin. J Physiol (Lond) 108:491–501

54. Peart WS (1954) Persistence of hypertension after removal of phaeochromocytoma, where excretion of adrenaline and noradrenaline is normal. In: Wolstenholme GEW, Cameron MP (eds) Ciba Foundation Symposium on Hypertension, Humoral and Neurogenic Factors. London, Churchill, pp 104–116

55. Pickering GW (1932) The vasomotor regulation of heat loss from the human skin in relation to external temperature. Heart 16:115–135

56. Polinsky RJ (1984) Central nervous system control of blood pressure. In: Weber MA, Mathias CJ (eds) Mild hypertension. Current controversies and new approaches. Steinkopff Darmstadt 11–23

57. Pourfois du Petit F (1727) Memoire dans lequel il est demonstre que les nerfs intercostaux fournissent des rameux qui portent des esprits dans les nerfs. Hist Acad Roy Sci Paris, p 1

58. Reid JL, Wing LMH, Mathias CJ, Frankel HL, Neill E (1977). The central hypotensive effect of clonidine: Studies in tetraplegic subjects. Clin Pharmacol Ther 21:375–381

59. Smirk FH (1959) High arterial pressure. Blackwell Scientific Publications, Oxford

60. Sjovall H, Jodal M, Lundgren O (1987) Sympathetic control of intestinal fluid and electrolyte transport. N Physiol Sci 2:214–217

61. Stella A, Golin R, Genovesi S, Zanchetti A (1986) Neural control of kidney function: Role of renorenal reflexes. In: Gloriosa N, Laragh JH, Rappelli A (eds) Renovascular Hypertension: Pathophysiology, Diagnosis and Treatment. Raven Press, New York, pp 187–194

62. Swales JD, Thurston H, Queiroz FP, Medina A (1972) Sodium balance during the development of experimental hypertension. J Lab Clin Med 80:539–547

63. Unwin RJ, Mathias CJ, Peart WS, Frankel HL (1986) Renal vascular responses to saralasin in conscious chemically denervated rabbits and patients with tetraplegia. Clin Experim Hypertension A8(6):919–939

64. Wallin BG, Fagius J (1988) Peripheral sympathetic neural activity in conscious humans. Ann Rev Physiol 50:565–576

65. Weinshilboum RM (1983) Biochemical genetics of catecholamines in humans. Mayo Clin Proc 58:319–330

66. Wilcox CS (1983) Body fluids and renal function in autonomic failure. In: Bannister R (ed) Autonomic Failure: a textbook of clinical disorders of the autonomic nervous system. Oxford University Press, Oxford pp 115–154

67. Zaimis E, Hanington E, (1969) A possible pharmacological approach to migraine. Lancet 3:298–300

68. Zimmerman BG (1981) Adrenergic facilitation by angiotensin: does it serve a physiological function? Clin Sci 60:343–348

Authors' address:
Dr. C. J. Mathias
Pickering Unit,
Department of Medicine
St Mary's Hospital,
Praed Street,
London W2 1NY.

# Concluding remarks

A. Zanchetti

Istituto di Clinica Medica Generale e Terapia Medica, University of Milan, and Centro Fisiologia Clinica e Ipertensione, Ospedale Maggiore, Milan, Italy

It is indeed a great honour to be asked to close this symposium in honour of Professor Sir Stanley Peart. Why should I have been asked? I am not among those who have been lucky enough to have passed through the Medical Unit at St. Mary's as members of the staff or as investigators. Nor is my English the most fluent one among those attending this meeting. Perhaps the reason is that I have known and admired Stan Peart for so many years. When I first met him, it was at the first International Symposium on Hypertension I attended, organized by Jan Brod in 1960 in Prague. Stan was then greatly admired because of his recent description of the amino-acid sequence of angiotensin and for developing sophisticated but laborious renin assays.

A few weeks after Prague, I again met Stan at the Ciba symposium organized by Franz Reubi and Paul Cottier in Berne, where Pickering and Platt crossed swords about the nature of essential hypertension, a knight against a baronet, the knight's sword being Sir George's well-known stick.

During the early 1960's, interest was growing in renovascular hypertension, as this was the classical, established experimental model of hypertension, and because of the clinical description of an increasing number of cases of this type of secondary hypertension. Renin assays were gradually becoming easier, although we did not yet foresee the era of the radioimmunoassays, and great expectations were nurtured that more frequent measurement of renin would have made differential diagnosis simpler.

In 1965, a second Ciba symposium was organized, this time by Cesare Bartorelli in Siena, and this was when I had my first training in organizing a meeting, having nobody less than Franz Gross as a teacher and as a German controller. At that meeting Stan Peart was invited to discuss the diagnosis of renovascular hypertension. As usual, with his critical judgement, Stan proceeded to show how often excessive expectations are eluded by data.

I have another document from the Siena symposium that was never printed, but I think it is appropriate to show it here. Perhaps Stan's happy excitement is not as interesting as Peggy's compassionate look (Fig. 1)!

I cannot mention all the occasions I have subsequently met Stan and learnt from him. As this is a satellite to a meeting held in Milan, I am proud to remember that Stan attended the very first ISH meeting held in Milan, in 1972. On that occasion, he presented the design of the MRC trial on mild hypertension. It is not meaningless, I believe, that it was on what has been learnt in the 15 years of this trial that Stan has based his contribution for the closing session of the Third European Meeting on Hypertension. He was the second of the wise men in the panel, and as you know, the

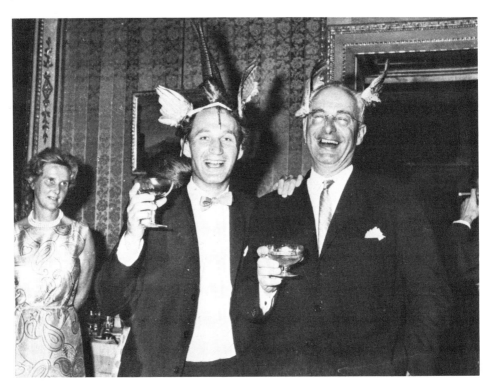

second wise man carries the incense. Stan has never used incense to praise or honour anybody, but rather – I suspect – to make smoke and incense somebody. At a time when many experts are urging treatment and even preaching overtreatment, he has not denied his old links with Sir George Pickering, nor has he forgotten Sir George's aphorism "There is no evidence that antihypertensive drugs prolong life – though no doubt it seems longer". Rather than any extreme position, he has recommended the value of investigation before any decision on treatment is taken.

*Investigation* is an appropriate word to stress at the end of these few words of tribute. The fact that Stan has used the word *investigation* instead of diagnostic procedures, I think is an indication of an approach, the approach that justifies the title and the outline of this tribute.

Diagnosis is simply the application to the individual of investigation into the mechanisms and signs of disease. Because of the wide and brilliant use of this approach, Sir Stanley Peart has enormously contributed to the improvement of the practice of medicine and to medical research. I remember the status of medical practice and research in hypertension in the early 1950s when Stan started his work, because I entered the field only a few years after him.

Today's activities and interest in the field have been documented in one way, by the huge attendance, the large participation in a European meeting such as the one in Milan. The contributions that Stan Peart has given personally or has promoted and triggered through the work of his students, by enlightening their minds or training their hands, have led to a widening of the experimental approach to hypertension that is witnessed in the scientific programme of this symposium volume, which could not have been envisaged 30 years ago.

Stan has provided all of us who work on hypertension with new concepts and he leaves these concepts to us with the hope, I am sure, that we are not accepting them, as they stand, but are soon going to challenge them – unless he is going to challenge and dispute them himself.

Authors' address:
Professor A. Zanchetti
Centro di Fisiologia
Clinica e Ipertensione
Ospedale Maggiore
Univ. di Milano
Via F. Sforza 35
20122 Milan, Italy

# Professional and bibliography

| | |
|---|---|
| **Name** | Sir [William] Stanley Peart |
| **Date of birth** | 31st March 1922 |
| **Nationality** | British |
| **Qualifications** | MB, BS (London), March 1945 |
| | MD (London), December 1949 |
| | FRCP (London), 1958 |
| **Academic distinctions** | Fellow of the Royal Society (1969) |
| | Stouffer Prize (1968) |
| | Membre honoraire étranger de l'Académic royale de Médecine de Belgique (1984) |
| | Honorary Member of the Association of American Physicians (1986) |

## Past appointments

Resident posts at St. Mary's Hospital, London, 1945–1946

Medical Research Council Studentship, Department of Pharmacology, Edinburgh University, 1946–1948

Medical Specialist, RAF Hospital, Ely (Rank: Squadron Leader), 1948–1950

Lecturer in Medicine, Medical Unit, St. Mary's Hospital, London, 1950–1953

Research Fellow, National Institute for Medical Research, Mill Hill, London, 1953–1955

Senior Lecturer in Medicine, Medical Unit, St. Mary's Hospital, London, 1955–1956

Professor of Medicine, University of London, at St. Mary's Hospital, London, 1956–1987

## Positions held in scientific societies

*Past*

Member, Medical Research Council
Member, Advisory Board for the Research Councils

**Publications**

Gaddum JH, Peart WS, Vogt M (1949) The estimation of adrenaline and allied substances in blood.
    J Physiol 108:467–481
Peart WS (1949) The nature of splenic sympathin. J Physiol 108:491–501
Hamilton M, Litchfield JW, Peart WS, Sowry GSC (1953) Phaeochromocytoma. Br Heart J
    15:241–249
Peart WS The control of vasomotor tone in hypertension
Peart WS (1954) Persistence of hypertension after the removal of phaeochromocytoma, where
    excretion of adrenaline and noradrenaline is normal. In: Ciba Foundation Symposium on
    Hypertension, Humoral and Neurogenic Factors. Churchill, London, pp 104–116
Peart WS The $\beta$-haloalkylamines
Davis P, Peart WS, van't Hoff W (1955) Malignant phaeochromocytoma with functioning metasta-
    ses. Lancet ii:274–275
Peart WS (1955) A new method of large scale preparation of hypertensin, with a note on its assay.
    Biochem J 59:300–302
Peart WS (1955) The purification of hypertensin. Biochem J 60:vi
Peart WS, Gordon DB, Cook WF, Pickering GW (1956) Distribution of renin in the rabbit kidney.
    Circulation 14:981–982
Peart WS (1956) Composition of a hypertensin peptide. Nature 177:132
Peart WS (1956) The isolation of a hypertensin. Biochem J 62:520–527
Elliott DF, Peart WS (1956) Amino acid sequence in a hypertensin. Nature 177:527–528
Pickering GW, Peart WS (1956) Hypertension. In: King EJ, Thompson RHS (eds) Topics in
    Chemical Pathology. Churchill, London
Peart WS (1956) Some substances antagonistic to the action of adrenaline and noradrenaline. In:
    Symposium on Hypotensive Drugs, and the Control of Vascular Tone in Hypertension: Co-
    ordinating Committee for Drug Action. Pergamon Press, London
Litchfield JW, Peart WS (1956) Phaeochromocytoma with normal excretion of adrenaline and
    noradrenaline. Lancet ii:1283–1284
Peart WS (1956) The clinical management of phaeochromocytoma. In: Symposium on the Clinical
    Management of Hypertension: Postgraduate Medical School of London, pp 90–95

Cook W, Gordon DB, Peart WS (1957) The location of renin in the rabbit kidney. J Physiol 135:46P–47P

Elliott DF, Peart WS (1957) The amino acid sequence in a hypertensin. Biochem J 65:246–254

Peart WS (1957–58) Some biochemical aspects of hypertension. In: Lectures on the Scientific Basis of Medicine, Vol 7. Athlone Press, p 182–202

Mowbray JF, Peart WS (1958) Some effects of noradrenaline and adrenaline on the thyroid. J Physiol (Lond) 143:12P

Peart WS, Sutton D (1958) Renal vein catheterisation and venography: a new technique. Lancet ii:817–818

Lever AF, Mowbray JF, Peart WS (1959) Blood flow and pressure after noradrenaline infusion. J Physiol (Lond) 146:43P–44P

Peart WS (1959) Renin and hypertensin. Ergebnisse Physiol 50:409–432

Peart WS (1959) A biased guide to renal hypertension. Arch Int Med 104:347–352

Peart WS, Robertson JIS, Andrews TM (1959) Facial flushing produced in patients with carcinoid syndrome by intravenous adrenaline and noradrenaline. Lancet ii:715–716

Peart WS (1959) Hypertension and the kidney. I. Clinical, pathological and functional disorders, especially in man. Br Med J ii:1353–1359

Peart WS (1959) Hypertension and the kidney. II. Experimental basis of renal hypertension. Br Med J ii:1421–1429

Mowbray JF, Peart WS (1960) Effects of noradrenaline and adrenaline on the thyroid. J Physiol (Lond) 151:261–271

Andrews TM, Peart WS, Robertson JIS (1960) The release of serotonin by intravenous adrenaline and noradrenaline. J Physiol (Lond) 155:8P–9P

Rob C, Peart WS (1960) Arterial auscultation. Lancet ii:219–220

Peart WS (1960) Angiotensin in experimental and clinical hypertension. In: Schachter M (ed) Polypeptides which affect Smooth Muscles and Blood Vessels: A Symposium. Pergamon Press, pp 122–136

Peart WS (1960) Possible relationship between salt metabolism and the angiotensin system. In: Bock KD, Cottier PT (eds) Essential Hypertension: An International Symposium. Springer-Verlag, pp 112–120

Peart WS (1960) Renal humoral factors in essential hypertension. In: The Pathogenesis of Essential Hypertension: Proceedings of the Prague Symposium. State Medical Publishing House, pp 418–429

Brown JJ, Owen K, Peart WS, Robertson JIS, Sutton D (1960) The diagnosis and treatment of renal artery stenosis. Br Med J ii:327–338

Peart WS (1961) High arterial pressure. In: Encyclopaedia "Life and Man", Les Editions de la Grange Bateliere, Paris

Peart WS, Brown JJ (1961) Effect of angiotensin (hypertensin or angiotonin) on urine flow and electrolyte excretion in hypertensive patients. Lancet i:28–29

Peart WS, Andrews TM, Robertson JIS (1961) Carcinoid syndrome: serotonin release induced with intravenous adrenaline and noradrenaline. Lancet i:577–578

Lever AF, Mowbray JF, Peart WS (1961) Blood flow and blood pressure after noradrenaline infusions. Clin Sci 21:69–74

Lever AF, Peart WS (1961) Pressor material in renal lymph. J Physiol (Lond) 159:35P–36P

Peart WS, Robertson JIS (1961) The effect of a serotonin antagonist (UML 491) in carcinoid disease. Lancet ii:1172–1174

Peart WS, Robertson JIS, Grahame-Smith DG (1961) Examination of the relationship of renin release to hypertension produced in the rabbit by renal artery constriction. Circulation Res 9:1171–1184

Peart WS (1961) The nature of renal hypertension. In: Fryer JH (ed) Hypertension and Coronary Artery Disease: Proceedings of a Symposium held in Chelmsford under the auspices of the Chelmsford Medical Society and the Mid-Essex Branch of the British Medical Association, 28–29 October. Pitman, London, pp 14–29

Brown JJ, Peart WS (1962) The effect of angiotensin on urine flow and electrolyte excretion in hypertensive patients. Clin Sci 22:1–17

Robertson JIS, Peart WS, Andrews TM (1962) The mechanism of facial flushes in the carcinoid syndrome. Quart J Med 31:103–123

Lever AF, Peart WS (1962) Renin and angiotensin-like activity in renal lymph. J Physiol (Lond) 160:548–563

Peart WS (1962) Drugs affecting the blood pressure and vasomotor tone. Ann Rev Pharmacol 2:251–268

Peart WS (1962) Hypertension and the kidney. In: Black DAK (ed) Renal disease. Blackwell, Oxford, pp 483–507

James VHT, Peart WS, Iles SD (1962) Steroid excretion in idiopathic hirsutism. J Endocr 24:463–470

Owen K, Peart WS (1962) Surgery of renal artery stenosis. In: Irvine WT (ed) Modern Trends in Surgery. Butterworths, London, pp 94–105

Peart WS (1962) Humoral factors in essential hypertension. Verhandl Dtsch Ges Kreislaufforschg 28:1–11

Peart WS, Porter KA, Robertson JIS, Sandler M, Baldock E (1963) Carcinoid syndrome due to pancreatic-duct neoplasm secreting 5-hydroxytryptophan and 5-hydroxytryptamine. Lancet i:239–243

Peart WS (1963) Sympathomimetic amines and angiotensin amide. Prescribers' J 3(1):7–9

Porter KA, Owen K, Mowbray JF, Thomson WB, Kenyon JR, Peart WS (1963) Obliterative vascular changes in four human kidney homotransplants. Br Med J ii:639–645

De Bono E, Lee G de J, Mottram FR, Pickering GW, Brown JJ, Keen H, Peart WS, Sanderson PH (1963) The action of angiotensin in man. Clin Sci 25:123–157

Peart WS (1963) The renal basis of hypertension. Biochemical Clinics, No 2, The Kidney, 267–274

Peart WS, MacMahon MT (1964) Clinical trial of 2-Guanidinomethyl (1,4) Benzodioxan (Compound 1003). Br Med J i:398–402

Peart WS (1964) Renal artery stenosis. In: Mackey WA, MacFarlane JA, Christian MS (eds) Arterial Surgery: Proceedings of the Conference at Law Hospital, Carluke. Pergamon Press, pp 27–40

Thomson WB, Buchanan AA, Doak PB, Peart WS (1964) Peritoneal dialysis. Br Med J i:932–935

Peart WS (1964) Hypertension and the kidney. Practitioner 193:14–26

Ellis CJ, Hamer DB, Hunt RW, Lever AF, Lever RS, Peart WS, Walker SM (1964) Medical investigation of retinal vascular occlusion. Br Med J ii:1093–1098

Brown JJ, Davies DL, Lever AF, Peart WS, Robertson JIS (1964) Plasma renin in a case of Conn's syndrome with fibrinoid lesions: use of spironolactone in treatment. Br Med J 2:1636–1637

Porter KA, Peart WS, Kenyon JR, Joseph NH, Hoehn RJ, Calne RY (1964) Rejection of kidney homotransplants. Ann NY Acad Sci 120:472–495

Peart WS (1965) The renin-angiotensin system. Pharmacol Rev 17:143–182

Peart WS (1965) Functional renal disorders in primary vascular disease. Renal Function: A Symposium. J Clin Path 18:564–567

Peart WS (1965) The carcinoid syndrome. In: Compston N (ed) Symposium on Advanced Medicine: Proceedings of a Conference held at the Royal College of Physicians of London, 16–20 November 1964. Pitman, London, pp 380–387

Peart WS (1965) Clinical and biochemical aspects of carcinoid tumours. In: Thackray AC, Avery Jones F (eds) The Small Intestine: A Symposium of the 5th Congress of the International Academy of Pathology. Blackwell, Oxford, pp 119–131

Mowbray JF, Cohen SL, Doak PB, Kenyon JR, Owen K, Percival A, Porter KA, Peart WS (1965) Human cadaveric renal transplantation: Report of twenty cases. Br Med J 2:1387–1394

Peart WS, Lloyd AM, Thatcher GN, Payne N, Stone N, Lever AF (1965) Purification of pig renin. Biochem J 96:31C

Peart WS (1965) The functions for renin and angiotensin. Recent Progr Hormone Res 21:73–118

Brown JJ, Davies DL, Lever AF, Peart WS, Robertson JIS (1965) Plasma concentration of renin in a patient with Conn's syndrome with fibrinoid lesions of the renal arterioles: the effect of treatment with spironolactone. J Endocr 33:279–293

Peart WS (1966) Catecholamines and hypertension. Pharmacol Rev 18:667–672

Peart WS (1966) Carcinoid tumours. Acta med scand 179 (suppl 445):371–376 [Also published as a book "In Honour of Jan Waldenström" on his 60th birthday, 17 April 1966]

Peart WS (1966) Diagnosis of renal artery stenosis. In: Gross F (ed) Antihypertensive Therapy, Principles and Practice: Proceedings of Symposium sponsored by CIBA held in Siena, 28 June– 3 July 1965. Springer-Verlag, Berlin/Heidelberg, pp 468–484

Peart WS, Lubash GD, Thatcher GN, Muiesan G (1966) Electrophoresis of pig and human renin. Biochim Biophys Acta 118:640–643

Peart WS, Lloyd AM, Thatcher GN, Lever AF, Payne N, Stone N (1966) Purification of pig renin. Biochem J 99:708–716

Peart WS (1966) Cadaveric renal transplantation. In: Losse H, Kienitz M (eds) Die Pyelonephritis. Georg Thieme Verlag, Stuttgart, pp 390–398

Lubash GD, Peart WS (1966) Purification of human renin. Biochim Biophys Acta 122:289–297

Peart WS (1967) The treatment of hypertension associated with renal artery stenosis. In: Engel A, Larsson T (eds) Stroke: Proceedings of Thule International Symposium held in Stockholm, 19–21 April 1966, sponsored by the Skandia Group. Nordiska Bokhandelns Forlag, Stockholm, pp 237–248

Peart WS (1967) Endocrine aspects of hypertension. In: Gardiner-Hill H (ed) Modern Trends in Endocrinology 3. Butterworths, London, pp 218–241

Porter KA, Dossetor JB, Marchioro TL, Peart WS, Rendall JM, Starzl TE, Terasaki PI (1967) Human renal transplants. I. Glomerular changes. Lab Invest 16:153–181

Peart WS (1967) Arterial hypertension. In: Beeson PB, McDermott W (eds) CECIL-LOEB Textbook of Medicine, Twelfth Edition. Saunders, Philadelphia, pp 657–666

Peart WS (1967) Pressor assays in the evaluation of renal hypertension. Proc 3rd Int Congr Nephrol, Washington 1966, Vol 3. Karger, Basel/New York, pp 140–151

Landon J, James VHT, Peart WS (1967) Cushing's syndrome associated with a corticotrophin producing bronchial neoplasm. Acta Endocr 56:321–332

Peart WS (1967) Hypertension and the kidney. In: Black DAK (ed) Renal Disease, Second Edition. Blackwell, Oxford, pp 638–664

Peart WS (1967) Renin and angiotensin. In: Gray CH, Bacharach AL (eds) Hormones in Blood, 2nd Edition. Academic Press, London/New York, pp 489–518

Lubash GD, Peart WS (1967) Determination of serum and plasma angiotensinase activity. Clin Chim Acta 17:445–447

Boyd GW, Landon J, Peart WS (1967) Radioimmunoassay for determining plasma levels of angiotensin II in man. Lancet 2:1002–1005

Boyd GW, Landon J, Peart WS (1968) Some problems encountered in the radioimmunoassay of circulating angiotensin II. In: Margoulies M (ed) Protein and Polypeptide Hormones, Part 2: Proceedings of the International Symposium, Liege, 19–25 May. Excerpta Medica Foundation, pp 365–369

Peart WS (1968) Renin and angiotensin. In: Astwood EB, Cassidy CE (eds) Clinical Endocrinology, Vol II. Grune and Stratton, New York, pp 778–788

Boyd GW, Peart WS (1968) The production of high-titre antibody against free angiotensin II. Lancet 2:129–133

Peart WS (1968) Aspects of cadaveric transplantation. Clin Chim Acta 22:91–93

Rappelli A, Peart WS (1968) Renal excretion of renin in the rat. Circulation Res 23:531–537

Pletka P, Cohen SL, Hulme B, Kenyon JR, Owen K, Thompson AE, Snell M, Mowbray JF, Porter KA, Leigh DA, Peart WS (1969) Cadaveric renal transplantation: an analysis of 65 cases. Lancet i:1–6

Fraser R, James VHT, Landon J, Peart WS, Rawson A, Giles CA, McKay AM (1968) Clinical and biochemical studies of a patient with a corticosterone-secreting adrenocortical tumour. Lancet ii:1116–1120

Peart WS (1968) Renal transplantation. In: Wrong O (ed) Fourth Symposium on Advanced Medicine: Proceedings of a Conference held at the Royal College of Physicians of London, 26 February–1 March. Pitman, Bath, pp 115–133

Boyd GW, Adamson AR, Fitz AE, Peart WS (1969) Radioimmunoassay determination of plasma-renin activity. Lancet i:213–218

Peart WS (1969) A history and review of the renin-angiotensin system. Proc R Soc B 173:317–325

Boyd GW, Landon J, Peart WS (1969) The radioimmunoassay of angiotensin II. Proc R Soc B 173:327–338

Peart WS, Boyd GW, James VHT, Macdonald GJ, Adamson AR (1969) Angiotensin and aldosterone. In: IVth International Congress of Nephrology, 22–27 June, Stockholm, Sweden, pp 141–143

Adamson AR, Grahame-Smith DG, Peart WS, Starr M (1969) Pharmacological blockade of carcinoid flushing provoked by catecholamines and alcohol. Lancet ii:293–297

Peart WS (1970) Cadaveric renal transplantation. In: Maxwell Anderson J (ed) The Biology and Surgery of Tissue Transplantation. Blackwell, Oxford/Edinburgh, pp 225–243

Peart WS, Boyd GW (1968) The radioimmunoassay of angiotensin I and II. In: Progress in Endocrinology: Proceedings of the Third International Congress of Endocrinology, held in Mexico, DF, 30 June–5 July. Excerpta Medica International Congress Series, No 184, pp 264–271

Boyd GW, Adamson AR, James VHT, Peart WS (1969) The rôle of the renin-angiotensin system in the control of aldosterone in man. Proc R Soc Med 62:1253–1254

Cuthbert MF, Peart WS (1970) Studies on the identity of a vascular permeability factor of renal origin. Clin Sci 38:309–325

Peart WS (1970) Hypertension. In: Thompson RHS, Wootton IDP (eds) Biochemical Disorders in Human Disease, Third Edition. Churchill, London, pp 233–254

Peart WS (1970) Death of the Professor of Medicine. Lancet i:401–402

Peart WS (1970) A University Hospital: President's Address, Section of Experimental Medicine and Therapeutics. Proc R Soc Med 63:383–385

Louis WJ, Macdonald GJ, Renzini V, Boyd GW, Peart WS (1970) Renal-clip hypertension in rabbits immunised against angiotensin II. Lancet i:333–335

Finberg JPM, Peart WS (1970) Renal tubular flow dynamics during angiotensin diuresis in the rat. Br J Pharmacol 39:357–372

Finberg JPM, Peart WS (1970) Function of smooth muscle of the rat renal pelvis – response of the isolated pelvis muscle to angiotensin and some other substances. Br J Pharmacol 39:373–381

Finberg JPM, Peart WS (1970) Intrarenal blood flow distribution in the rat, and the effect of angiotensin, noradrenaline and vasopressin. J Physiol (Lond) 209:21P–22P

Peart WS (1970) Renin and angiotensin in relation to aldosterone. Am J Clin Path 54:324–330

Peart WS (1970) Medicinal chemistry for the next decade. In: Ellis GP, West GB (eds) Progress in Medicinal Chemistry, Vol 7, Part 2. Butterworths, London, pp 215–228

Macdonald GJ, Louis WJ, Renzini V, Boyd GW, Peart WS (1970) Renal-clip hypertension in rabbits immunized against angiotensin II. Circulation Res 27:197–211

Pessina AC, Hulme B, Rappelli A, Peart WS (1970) Renin excretion in patients with renal disease. Circulation Res 27:891–899

Adamson AR, Grahame-Smith DG, Peart WS, Starr M (1971) Pharmacological blockade of carcinoid flushing provoked by catecholamines and alcohol. Am Heart J 81:141–142

Peart WS (1971) Renin-angiotensin system in hypertensive disease. In: Fisher JW (ed) Kidney Hormones. Academic Press, London, pp 217–242

Peart WS (1971) Arterial hypertension. In: Beeson PB, McDermott W (eds) CECIL-LOEB Textbook of Medicine, Thirteenth Edition. Saunders, Philadelphia, pp 1050–1062

Boyd GW, Peart WS (1971) The relationship between angiotensin and aldosterone. In: Levine R, Luft R (eds) Advances in Metabolic Disorders, Vol 5. Academic Press, New York, pp 77–117

Peart WS (1971) Renin and renal hypertension. In: Klutsch K, Wollheim E, Holtmeier H-J (eds) Die Niere im Kreislauf, 9. Internationales Symposon der Deutschen Gesellschaft für Fortschritte auf dem Gebiet der Inneren Medizin, Würzburg, April 1970. Georg Thieme Verlag, Stuttgart, pp 166–170

Pessina AC, Peart WS (1972) Renin induced proteinuria and the effects of adrenalectomy. I. Haemodynamic changes in relation to function. Proc R Soc Lond B 180:43–60

Pessina AC, Hulme B, Peart WS (1972) Renin induced proteinuria and the effects of adrenalectomy. II. Morphology in relation to function. Proc R Soc Lond B 180:61–71

Pessina AC, Peart WS (1972) The effects of renin and adrenalectomy on blood distribution and capillary permeability. Proc R Soc Lond B 180:73–85

Finberg JPM, Peart WS (1972) The effect of angiotensin, noradrenaline and vasopressin on blood flow distribution in the rat kidney. J Physiol (Lond) 220:229–242

Boyd GW, Adamson AR, Arnold M, James VHT, Peart WS (1972) The rôle of angiotensin II in the control of aldosterone in man. Clin Sci 42:91–104

Macdonald GJ, Boyd GW, Peart WS (1972) Renal hypertension and angiotensin antibodies. Am Heart J 83:137–139

Lowenstein J, Boyd GW, Rippon AE, James VHT, Peart WS (1972) Increased aldosterone in response to sodium deficiency in the angiotensin II-immunized rabbit. In: Hypertension 1972. Springer-Verlag, Berlin/Heidelberg, pp 481–489

Boyd GW, Jones MBS, Peart WS (1972) The radioimmunoassay of angiotensin II and plasma renin activity in human hypertension. In: Hypertension 1972. Springer-Verlag, Berlin/Heidelberg, pp 583–591

Abbott EC, James VHT, Parker RA, Peart WS, Fraser R (1972) The effect of a sulphated mucopolysaccharide (RO1-8307) on adrenal and kidney morphology and function in the rat. Hormones 3:129–143

Hulme B, Kenyon JR, Owen K, Snell M, Mowbray JF, Porter KA, Starkie SJ, Muras H, Peart WS (1972) Renal transplantation in children. Analysis of 25 consecutive transplants in 19 recipients. Arch Dis Childhood 47 (No 254):486–494

Hulme B, Snell ME, Kenyon JR, Owen K, Peart WS (1972) Kidney preservation by surface cooling: analysis of 130 transplants. Br Med J 4:139–141

Peart WS (1972) Hypertension and the kidney. In: Black, Sir Douglas (ed) Renal Disease, Third Edition. Blackwell, Oxford, pp 705–737

Peart WS (1973) The kideny and secretion of aldosterone. In: Actualités Néphrologiques de l'Hôpital Necker. Flammarion Médecine-Sciences, Paris, pp 301–306. [Reproduced in Advances in Nephrology 3:289–295, 1974]

Richards P, Jones MBS, Peart WS (1973) Periodic hypokalaemic paralysis, adrenal adenoma, and normal colonic transport of sodium and potassium. Gut 14:478–484

Vandongen R, Peart WS, Boyd GW (1973) Adrenergic stimulation of renin secretion in the isolated perfused rat kidney. Circulation Res 32:290–296

Peart WS (1973) Methods of extraction and purification of peptide hormones. 2. From plasma. In: Berson SA, Yalow RS (eds) Methods in Investigative and Diagnostic Endocrinology, Vol 2A. North-Holland Publishing Co, Amsterdam, pp 10–19

Peart WS (1973) Angiotensin I and II. I. Purification and biochemical characterization. In: Berson SA, Yalow RS (eds) Methods in Investigative and Diagnostic Endocrinology, Vol 2B. North-Holland Publishing Co, Amsterdam, pp 1145–1149

Peart WS (1973) The organization of a multi-centre randomized control therapeutic trial for mild to moderate hypertension. Clin Sci Mol Med 45:67s–70s

Peart WS (1973) Results of medical versus surgical treatment of renovascular hypertension. Clin Sci Mol Med 45:89s–93s

Peart WS (1973) Renal hypertension: does it relate to essential hypertension? In: Onesti G, Kim KE, Moyer JH (eds) Hypertension: Mechanisms and Management: Twenty-Sixth Hahnemann Symposium. Grune and Stratton, New York, pp 727–740

Peart WS (1973) Renal hypertension. In: Sambhi MP (ed) Mechanisms of Hypertension: Proceedings of an International Workshop Conference held in Los Angeles, 7–9 March, International Congress Series No 302. Excerpta Medica, Amsterdam, pp 59–64

Peart WS (1974) The kidney and the secretion of aldosterone. Adv Nephrol 3:289–295

Boyd GW, Peart WS (1974) Angiotensin immunoassay. In: Page IH, Bumpus FM (eds) Angiotensin, Handb Exp Pharm XXXVII. Springer-Verlag, Berlin/Heidelberg/New York, pp 211–226

Vandongen R, Peart WS (1974) Calcium dependence of the inhibitory effect of angiotensin on renin secretion in the isolated perfused kidney of the rat. Br J Pharmacol 50:125–129

Efstratopoulos AD, Peart WS, Wilson GA (1974) The effect of aldosterone on colonic potential difference and renal electrolyte excretion in normal man. Clin Sci Mol Med 46:489–499

Peart WS (1973) Medical research is too important to be left to the researchers! Lecture given at the Royal Institution, Albemarle Street, London, W1, on 18 October, to mark the 25th Anniversary of the foundation of the Glaxo Volume

Vandongen R, Peart WS, Boyd GW (1974) Effect of angiotensin II and its nonpressor derivatives on renin secretion. Am J Physiol 226:227–282

Efstratopoulos AD, Peart WS, Wilson GA (1974) The effect of aldosterone on colonic potential difference and renal electrolyte excretion in normal man. Clin Sci Mol Med 46:489–499

Cohen SL, Gorchein A, Hayward JA, Kennerley Bankes JL, Petrie A, Porter KA, Peart WS (1974) Pingueculae – an association with renal failure. Quart J Med, New Series, 43:281–291

Besterman E, Bromley LL, Peart WS (1974) An intrapericardial phaeochromocytoma. Br Heart J 36:318–320

Goodwin TJ, James VHT, Peart WS (1974) The control of aldosterone secretion in nephrectomized man. Clin Sci Mol Med 47:235–248

Vandongen R, Peart WS (1974) The inhibition of renin secretion by alpha-adrenergic stimulation in the isolated rat kidney. Clin Sci Mol Med 47:471–479

Peart WS (1974) Impediments to research in hospitals. In: Symposium on Constraints on the Advance of Medicine: Proceedings of the Royal Society of Medicine, Vol 67 (No 12, Part 2, Symp No 15):pp 1285–1287

Ferriss JB, Brown JJ, Fraser R, Haywood E, Davies DL, Kay AW, Lever AF, Robertson JIS, Owen K, Peart WS (1975) Results of adrenal surgery in patients with hypertension, aldosterone excess, and low plasma renin concentration. Br Med J 1:135–138

Efstratopoulos AD, Peart WS (1975) Effect of single and combined infusions of angiotensin II and aldosterone on colonic potential difference, blood pressure and renal function, in patients with adrenal deficiency. Clin Sci Mol Med 48:219–226

Peart WS (1975) Renin-angiotensin system. New Engl J Med 292:302–306

Peart WS, Quesada T, Tenyi I (1975) The effects of cyclic adenosine 3′,5′-monophosphate and guanosine 3′,5′-monophosphate and theophylline on renin secretion in the isolated perfused kidney of the rat. Br J Pharmacol 54:55–60

Peart WS (1975) Arterial hypertension. In: Beeson PB, McDermott W (eds) Textbook of Medicine, Fourteenth Edition. Saunders, Philadelphia/London/Toronto, pp 981–992

Logan AG, Tenyi I, Quesada T, Peart WS, Breathnach AS, Martin BGH (1975) Blockade of renin release by lanthanum. Clin Sci Mol Med 48:31s–32s

Peart WS, Pessina AC (1975) The mechanism of acute renal ischaemia caused by adrenalectomy in the rat. J Physiol (Lond) 250:23–37

Lennane RJ, Peart WS, Shaw J (1975) Adrenergic influences on the electrical potential across the colonic mucosa of the rabbit. J Physiol (Lond) 250:367–372

Mathias CJ, Christensen NJ, Corbett JL, Frankel HL, Goodwin TJ, Peart WS (1975) Plasma catecholamines, plasma renin activity and plasma aldosterone in tetraplegic man, horizontal and tilted. Clin Sci Mol Med 49:291–299

Lennane RJ, Peart WS, Carey RM, Shaw J (1975) A comparison of natriuresis after oral and intravenous sodium loading in sodium-depleted rabbits: evidence for a gastrointestinal or portal monitor of sodium intake. Clin Sci Mol Med 49:433–436

Lennane RJ, Carey RM, Goodwin TJ, Peart WS (1975) A comparison of natriuresis after oral and intravenous sodium loading in sodium-depleted man: evidence for a gastrointestinal or portal monitor of sodium intake. Clin Sci Mol Med 49:437–440

Peart WS (1975) The place of renin in the mechanism of hypertension in chronic renal disease. Clin Nephrol 4:138–143

Macdonald GJ, Boyd GW, Peart WS (1975) Effect of the angiotensin II blocker 1-sar-8-ala-angiotensin II on renal artery clip hypertension in the rat. Circulation Res 37:640–646

Macdonald GJ, Boyd GW, Peart WS (1975) The effect of an angiotensin blocker, sarcosyl[1]-alanyl[8]-angiotensin II (P113) on two kidney hypertension in the rat. Clin Exp Pharmacol Physiol, Suppl 2, 89–91

Peart WS (1976) The renin-angiotensin system. In: Parsons JA (ed) Peptide Hormones. Macmillan, London/Basingstoke, pp 179–196

Lennane RJ, Stockigt J, Peart WS (1976) The effect of active immunization against aldosterone on the colonic potential response and sodium excretion in rabbits. Clin Sci Mol Med 50:545–549

Lancaster R, Goodwin TJ, Peart WS (1976) The effect of pindolol on plasma renin activity and blood pressure in hypertensive patients. Br J Clin Pharmacol 3:453–460

Peart WS (1976) Advances in renal endocrinology. Proc 6th Int Congr Nephrol, Florence 1975. Karger, Basel, pp 38–48

Peart WS (1976) The problems of morbidity and therapy in borderline hypertension. Schweiz Med Wschr 106:1706–1711

Britton KE, Goodwin TJ, Peart WS, Snell ME (1976) Adrenal aldosterone-producing adenoma: use of colonic potential in diagnosis and subtraction scanning technique for localisation. Br Med J 2:11–14

Logan AG, Tenyi I, Peart WS, Breathnach AS, Martin BGH (1977) The effect of lanthanum on renin secretion and renal vasoconstriction. Proc R Soc Lond B 195:327–342

Peart WS, Quesada T, Tenyi I (1977) The effects of EDTA and EGTA on renin secretion. Br J Pharmacol 59:247–252

Fynn M, Onomakpome N, Peart WS (1977) The effects of ionophores (A23187 and RO2-2985) on renin secretion and renal vasoconstriction. Proc R Soc Lond B 199:199–212

Peart WS (1977) The kidney as an endocrine organ. Lancet ii:543–548

Peart WS (1977) Generalities on hypertension. In: Genest J, Koiw E, Kuchel O (eds) Hypertension. McGraw-Hill, New York, pp 3–9

Peart WS (1977) Personal views on mechanisms of hypertension. In: Genest J, Koiw E, Kuchel O (eds) Hypertension. McGraw-Hill, New York, pp 588–597

Medical Research Council Working Party on Mild Hypertension (Chairman: Professor WS Peart) (1977) Randomised controlled trial of treatment for mild hypertension: design and pilot trial. Br Med J 1:1437–1440

Peart WS (1978) Renin release. Gen Pharmac 9:65–72

Peart WS (1978) Mild hypertension. In: Weatherall DJ (ed) Advanced Medicine 14. Pitman, Tunbridge Wells, pp 87–98

Peart WS (1978) Intra-renal factors in renin release. Contr Nephrol, Vol 12. Karger, Basel, pp 5–15

Gordon D, James VHT, Peart WS, Wilson GA (1978) Changes in urinary aldosterone excretion and plasma renin activity in response to dietary sodium chloride deprivation in man. J Physiol (Lond) 280:43P–44P

Williams BI, Peart WS (1978) Effects of posture on the intraocular pressure of patients with retinal vein obstruction. Br J Ophthalmol 62:688–693

Peart WS (1978) Renin 1978. Johns Hopkins Med J 143:193–206

Peart WS (1979) Editorial: Research in psychiatry: a view from general medicine. Psychol Med 9:205–206

Gordon D, Peart WS, Wolcox CS (1979) Requirement of the adrenergic nervous system for conservation of sodium by the rabbit kidney. J Physiol (Lond) 293:24P

Sagnella G, Peart WS (1979) Studies on the isolation and properties of renin granules from the rat kidney cortex. Biochem J 182:301–309

Gordon D, Peart WS (1979) Sodium excretion in man, and adaptation to a low-sodium diet: effect of intravenous sodium chloride. Clin Sci 57:225–231

Peart WS (1979) Humors and hormones. The Harvey Lectures, Series 73. Academic Press, New York, pp 259–290

James VHT, Lightman SL, Linsell C, Mullen PE, Peart WS (1979) The influence of the rapid eye movement phase of sleep on plasma renin activity in man. J Physiol (Lond) 295:69P

Williams BI, Peart WS (1979) Retinal vein obstruction and intraocular pressure: abnormal postural response independent of facility of outflow. Br J Ophthalmol 63:805–807

Sever PS, Peart WS, Meade TW, Davies IB, Gordon D (1979) Ethnic differences in blood pressure with observations on noradrenaline and renin. 1. A working population. Clin Exp Hypertension 1:733–744

Sever PS, Peart WS, Davies IB, Tunbridge RDG, Gordon D (1979) Ethnic differences in blood pressure with observations on noradrenaline and renin. 2. A hospital hypertensive population. Clin Exp Hypertension 1:745–760

Kapoor A, Porter KA, Mowbray JF, Peart WS (1980) Significance of haematuria in hypertensive patients. Lancet 1:231–232

Heller RF, Robinson N, Peart WS (1980) Value of blood pressure measurement in relatives of hypertensive patients. Lancet 1:1206–1208

Peart WS (1980) Concepts in hypertension. J Royal Coll Phys of Lond 14:141–152

Lightman SL, James VHT, Linsell C, Mullen PE, Peart WS (1980) Influence of Zeitgebers and nocturnal activity of the central nervous system on plasma levels and relationships of renin activity, aldosterone and cortisol. J Endocrinol 85:16P

Sever PS, Gordon D, Peart WS, Beighton P (1980) Blood pressure and its correlates in urban and tribal Africa. Lancet 2:60–64

Mullen PE, James VHT, Lightman SL, Linsell C, Peart WS (1980) A relationship between plasma renin activity and the rapid eye movement phase of sleep in man. J Clin Endocr Metab 50:466–469

Peart WS (1980) The Pharmaceutical Industry: research and responsibility. Lancet 2:465–466

Mathias CJ, Christensen NJ, Frankel HL, Peart WS (1980) Renin release during head-up tilt occurs independently of sympathetic nervous activity in tetraplegic man. Clin Sci 59:251–256

Sagnella GA, Caldwell PRB, Peart WS (1980) Subcellular distribution of low- and high-molecular-weight renin and its relation to a renin inhibitor in pig renal cortex. Clin Sci 59:337–345

Williams BI, Peart WS, Letley E (1980) Abnormal intraocular pressure control in systemic hypertension and diabetes mellitus. Br J Ophthalmol 64:845–851

Sagnella G, Price R, Peart WS (1980) Subcellular distribution and storage form of rat renal renin. Hypertension 2:595–603

Peart WS (1980) The influence of various neurological defects on the release of renin in normal man. In: Case DB, Sonnenblick EH, Laragh JH (eds) Captopril and Hypertension. Plenum Medical Book Co, New York/London, pp 39–56

Forsling ML, Lightman S, Moss S, Peart WS (1980) The water diuresis in response to dietary sodium deprivation in patients with ileostomies. J Physiol (Lond) 306:36P–37P

Gordon D, James VHT, Moss S, Peart WS, Roddis SA (1980) Adaptation to a low-sodium diet in subjects with ileostomies: changes in renin and aldosterone, and in the electrolyte composition of urine and ileal fluid. J Physiol (Lond) 306:41P

Gordon D, Peart WS, Roddis SA, Unwin RJ (1980) Renal function during pentagastrin infusion in conscious rabbits. J Physiol (Lond) 310:40P–41P

Peart WS, Sever PS, Swales JD, Tarazi RC (1980) Slide Atlas of Hypertension, sponsored by the International Society of Hypertension, produced and published by Gower Medical Publishing Ltd

Wilcox CS, Lewis PS, Peart WS, Sever PS, Osikowska BA, Suddle SAJ, Bluhm MM, Veall N, Lancaster R (1981) Renal function, body fluid volumes, renin, aldosterone, and noradrenaline during treatment of hypertension with Pindolol. J Cardiovasc Pharmacol 3:598–611

Wilcox CS, Lewis PS, Sever PS, Peart WS (1981) The actions of saralasin on the renal circulation of man and dog; evidence for a sympathetic neural component to vasoconstriction. Eur J Clin Invest 11:77–83

Moss S, Gordon D, Forsling ML, Peart WS, James VHT, Roddis SA (1981) Water and electrolyte composition of urine and ileal fluid and its relationship to renin and aldosterone during dietary sodium deprivation in patients with ileostomies. Clin Sci 61:407–415

Sagnella GA, Peart WS (1981) Properties of a renin inhibitor isolated from the pig kidney cortex. Clin Sci 60:639–651

Peart WS (1981) Advice from a not so young medical scientist. Clin Sci 61:364–368

Williams BI, Gordon D, Peart WS (1981) Abnormal variability of intraocular pressure and systemic arterial blood pressure in diabetes, hypertension, and retinal venous occlusion. Lancet 2:1255–1257

Peart WS (1981) The problem of treatment in mild hypertension. Clin Sci 61:403s–411s

Peart WS, Roddis SA, Unwin RJ (1981) In vivo evidence for renal tubular NaCa counter transport. J Physiol (Lond) 320:64P–65P

Frankel HL, Mathias CJ, Peart WS, Unwin RJ (1981) Saralasin-induced renal vasoconstriction is due to intrinsic angiotensin-II activity. J Physiol (Lond) 319:72P–73P

Peart WS (1981) Future prospects in hypertension research. In: Yu PN, Goodwin JF (eds) Progress in Cardiology. Lea & Febiger, Philadelphia, pp 150–156

Khaw KT, Peart WS (1982) Blood pressure and contraceptive use. Br Med J 285:403–407

Peart WS (1982) The problem of treatment of mild hypertension. Br J Clin Pharmacol 13:87–90

Frankel HL, Mathias CJ, Peart WS, Unwin RJ (1982) Indomethacin inhibits renin release to tilt, isoprenaline and frusemide in tetraplegic subjects. J Physiol (Lond) 325:62P

Calam J, Dimaline R, Peart WS, Unwin RJ (1982) Vasoactive intestinal polypeptide (VIP) and renin release in the conscious rabbit. J Physiol (Lond) 329:66P

Calam J, Peart WS, Singh J, Unwin RJ (1982) Renal function during vasoactive intestinal polypeptide infusion in man. J Physiol (Lond) 332:96P

Peart WS (1982) Renin-angiotensin system. Quart J Exp Physiol 67:401–406

McMichael J, Peart WS (1982) George White Pickering, 1904–1980, Elected F.R.S. 1960. Biographical Memoirs of Fellows of the Royal Society 28:431–449

Meade TW, Imeson JD, Gordon D, Peart WS (1983) The epidemiology of plasma renin. Clin Sci 64:273–280

Mathias CJ, Wilkinson A, Lewis PS, Peart WS, Sever PS, Snell ME (1983) Clonidine lowers blood pressure independently of renin suppression in patients with unilateral renal artery stenosis. Chest 83S:357S–359S

Calam J, Unwin R, Peart WS (1983) Neurotensin stimulates defaecation. Lancet 1:737–738

Peart WS (1983) Rebirth of the Professor of Medicine. Lancet 1:810–812

Calam J, Peart WS, Unwin RJ (1983) Renal effects of cholecystokinin octapeptide (CCK8) in the conscious rabbit. J Physiol (Lond) 334:122P

Bloom SR, Peart WS, Unwin RJ (1983) Neurotensin and antinatriuresis in the conscious rabbit. Br J Pharmacol 79:15–18

Peart WS (1983) General review of hypertension. In: Genest J, Kuchel O, Hamet P, Cantin M (eds) Hypertension, Physiopathology and Treatment: Second Edition. McGraw-Hill, New York, pp 3–14

Calam J, Dimaline R, Peart WS, Unwin R (1983) Studies on the renin response to vasoactive intestinal polypeptide (VIP) in the conscious rabbit. Br J Pharmacol 80:13–15

Peart WS, Unwin RJ (1983) Effects of substance P (SP) on renal function in conscious rabbits. J Physiol (Lond) 343:51P

Dimaline R, Peart WS, Unwin RJ (1983) Effects of vasoactive intestinal polypeptide (VIP) on renal function and plasma renin activity in the conscious rabbit. J Physiol (Lond) 344:379–388

Taylor GM, Peart WS (1983) The subcellular distribution and storage form of renin in human kidney cortex. J Hypertension 1:277–284

Calam J, Dimaline R, Peart WS, Singh J, Unwin RJ (1983) Effects of vasoactive intestinal polypeptide on renal function in man. J Physiol (Lond) 345:469–475

Snell ME, Lawrence R, Sutton D, Sever PS, Peart WS (1983) Advances in the techniques of localisation of adrenal tumours and their influence on the surgical approach to the tumour. Br J Urol 55:617–621

Peart WS, Sever PS, Swales JD, Tarazi RC (1984) Hypertension, Illustrated. Gower Medical Publishing Ltd, London

Mathias CJ, Wilkinson AH, Pike FA, Sever PS, Peart WS (1983) Clonidine in unilateral renal artery stenosis and unilateral renal parenchymal disease – similar antihypertensive but different renin suppressive effects. J Hypertension 1 (suppl 2):123–125

Mathias CJ, Unwin RJ, Pike FA, Frankel HL, Sever PS, Peart WS (1984) The immediate pressor response to saralasin in man: evidence against sympathetic activation and for intrinsic angiotensin II-like myotropism. Clin Sci 66:517–524

Peart WS (1984) Some neurological aspects of blood pressure control. In: Weber MA, Mathias CJ (eds) Mild hypertension – current controversies and new approaches: Proceedings of the International Titisee Workshop, 13–15 October 1983. Steinkopff, Darmstadt, pp 1–7

Mathias CJ, Peart WS, Carron DB, Hemingway AP, Allison DJ (1984) Therapeutic venous infarction of an aldosterone producing adenoma (Conn's tumour). Br Med J 288:1416–1417

Calam J, Peart WS, Reed T, Thom S, Unwin RJ (1984) The influence of indomethacin and DL-propranolol on the cardiovascular and renin responses to vasoactive intestinal polypeptide (VIP) in man. J Physiol (Lond) 358:121P

May CN, Peart WS (1984) The rôle of calcium in the control of renin release. J Hypertension 2 (suppl 3):243–245

Poulter N, Khaw KT, Hopwood BEC, Mugambi M, Peart WS, Rose G, Sever PS (1984) Blood pressure and its correlates in an African tribe in urban and rural environments. J Epidemiol Community Health 38:181–185

Poulter N, Khaw KT, Hopwood BEC, Mugambi M, Peart WS, Rose G, Sever PS (1984) Blood pressure and associated factors in a rural Kenyan community. Hypertension 6:810–813

Pulter N, Khaw KT, Hopwood BEC, Mugambi M, Peart WS, Sever PS (1984) Salt and blood pressure in various populations. J Cardiovasc Pharmacol 6:S197–S203

May CN, Peart WS (1985) Effect on the calcium agonist BAY-K-8644 on in vitro renin release from rat kidney cortex. J Physiol (Lond) 360:56P

Unwin RJ, Moss S, Peart WS, Wadsworth J (1985) Renal adaptation and gut hormone release during sodium restriction in ileostomized man. Clin Sci 69:299–308

Medical Research Council Working Party on Mild Hypertension (Chairman: Professor Sir Stanley Peart) (1985) MRC trial of treatment of mild hypertension: principal results. Br Med J 291:97–104

Wilcox CS, Roddis S, Peart WS, Gordon D, Lewis GP (1985) Intrarenal prostaglandin release: effects of arachidonic acid and hyperchloremia. Kidney Int 28:43–50

Peart S (1985) Role of drugs modifying sympathetic nervous activity, in the treatment of hypertension. J Hypertension 3 (suppl): 51–55

Mathias CJ, Wilkinson AH, Stone FA, Peart S (1985) Cardiovascular and hormonal effects of clonidine in patients with essential hypertension and renal hypertension. J Hypertension 3 (suppl 4):S73–S75

Mathias CJ, Da Costa DF, Cleary JC, Peart S (1985) Naloxone does not affect the cardiovascular, sedative or neurohormonal effects of clonidine in normal and hypertensive man. J Hypertension 3 (suppl 4):S77–S79

Poulter NR, Khaw K, Hopwood BE, Mugambi M, Peart WS, Sever PS (1985) Determinants of blood pressure changes due to urbanization: a longitudinal study. J Hypertension 3 (suppl 3): S375–S377

Taylor GM, Peart WS, Porter KA, Zondek LH, Zondek T (1986) Concentration and molecular forms of active and inactive renin in human fetal kidney, amniotic fluid and adrenal gland: evidence for renin-angiotensin system hyperactivity in 2nd trimester of pregnancy. J Hypertension 4:121–129

Carmichael DJS, Mathias CJ, Snell ME, Peart S (1986) Detection and investigation of renal artery stenosis. Lancet 1:667–670

Taylor GM, Carmichael DJS, Peart WS (1986) Active and inactive renin in anephric man: a comparison of molecular weight studies with normal human plasma and the effect of a specific monoclonal anti-renin antibody. J Hypertension 4:703–712

Peart WS, Roddis SA, Unwin RJ (1986) Renal electrolyte excretion and renin release during calcium and parathormone infusions in conscious rabbits. J Physiol (Lond) 373:329–341

May CN, Peart WS (1986) Stimulation and suppression of renin release from incubations of rat renal cortex by factors affecting calcium flux. Br J Pharmacol 89:173–182

Unwin RJ, Mathias CJ, Peart WS, Frankel HL (1986) Renal vascular responses to saralasin in conscious chemically denervated rabbits and patients with tetraplegia. Clin and Exper Hyper – Theory and Practice A8(6):919–939

Medical Research Council Working Party on Mild Hypertension (Chairman: Professor Sir Stanley Peart) (1986) Course of blood pressure in mild hypertensives after withdrawal of long term antihypertensive treatment. Br Med J 293:988–992

Mathias CJ, Gooner JS, Peart WS (1986) Do neurogenic mechanisms maintain hypertension in renal artery stenosis? In: Gloriosa N, Laragh JH, Rappelli A (eds) Renovascular Hypertension: Pathophysiology, Diagnosis and Treatment. Raven Press, New York, pp 173–185

Mathias CJ, Kooner JS, Peart WS (1986) Neurogenic mechanisms and the maintenance of hypertension in patients with renal artery stenosis. Quart J Med (New Series) 61:1069–1070

Carmichael DJS, Few JD, Peart WS, Unwin RJ (1986) Changes in salivary aldosterone (SA) concentration during dietary sodium restriction in two healthy males. J Physiol (Lond) 377:71P

Carmichael DJS, Peart WS, Unwin RJ (1986) In vitro study of the relationship between whole blood $Ca^{2+}$ ion activity ($a_{Ca}$) and total plasma calcium concentration in rabbit and man. J Physiol (Lond) 381:21P

Carmichael DJS, Peart WS, Unwin RJ (1987) Renal tubular effects and changes in whole blood calcium ion activity ($a_{Ca}$) during calcium chloride ($CaCl_2$) infusion in man. J Physiol (Lond) 382:146P

Boulter M, Brink A, Mathias C, Peart S, Stevens J, Stewart G, Unwin R (1987) Unusual cranial and abdominal computed tomographic (CT) scan appearances in a case of systemic lupus erythematosus (SLE). Ann Rheum Dis 46:162–165

Kooner JS, Few JD, Mathias CJ, Peart WS (1987) Salivary aldosterone measurements in the diagnosis of primary hyperaldosteronism. Clin Sci 72 (suppl 16):14P–15P

Kooner JS, Mathias CJ, Peart WS (1987) Haemodynamic changes during clonidine-induced hypotension in human renal artery stenosis. Clin Sci 72 (suppl 16):18P

Unwin RJ, Reed T, Thom S, Calam J, Peart WS (1987) Effects of indomethacin and (±)-propranolol on the cardiovascular and renin responses to vasoactive intestinal polypeptide (VIP) infusion in man. Br J Clin Pharmac 23:523–528

Calam J, Gordon D, Peart WS, Taylor SA, Unwin RJ (1987) Renal effects of gastrin C-terminal tetrapeptide (as pentagastrin) and cholecystokinin octapeptide in conscious rabbit and man. Br J Pharmac 91:307–314

Unwin RJ, Calam J, Peart WS, Hanson C, Lee YC, Bloom SR (1987) Renal function during bovine neurotensin infusion in man. Regulatory Peptides 18:29–35

Peart S (1987) Problems in the treatment of hypertension. J Hypertension 5 (suppl 5)

Mathias CJ, Kooner JS, Peart WS (1987) Neurogenic components of hypertension in human renal artery stenosis. Clin Exp Hypertension – Theory and Practice A9 (suppl 1):293–306

Bannister R, Frankel HL, Kooner JS, Mathias CJ, Peart WS (1987) Recumbency induced diuresis in human subjects with autonomic failure and tetraplegia. J Physiol (Lond) 390:2068

Kooner JS; Da Costa DF, Frankel HL, Bannister RB, Peart WS, Mathias CJ (1987) Recumbency induces hypertension, diuresis and natriuresis in autonomic failure but diuresis alone in tetraplegia. J Hypertension 5 (suppl 5):327–329

Peart WS (1987) Results of M.R.C. (U.K.) trial of drug therapy for mild hypertension. Clin Invest Med

Kooner JS, Edge W, Frankel HL, Peart WS, Mathias CJ (1988) Haemodynamic action of clonidine in tetraplegia – effects at rest and during bladder stimulation. Paraplegia 26:200–203

Peart S (1988) Is discovery worth the pain? Conquest (Journal of the Research Defence Society), No 177, 1–10

Taylor GM, Cook HT, Sheffield EA, Hanson C, Peart WS (1988) Renin in blood vessels in human pulmonary tumors. An immunohistochemical and biochemical study. Am J Path 130:543–551

Medical Research Council Working Party on Mild Hypertension (Chairman: Professor Sir Stanley Peart) (1988) Coronary heart disease in the Medical Research Council trial of treatment of mild hypertension. Br Heart J 59:364–378

Medical Research Council Working Party on Mild Hypertension (Chairman: Professor Sir Stanley Peart) (1988) Stroke and coronary heart disease in mild hypertension: risk factors and the value of treatment. Br Med J 296:1565–1570

# After-dinner speech

D. G. Grahame-Smith

Stan and Peggy, ladies and gentlemen, Peter Sever rang me up a few months ago and afforded me one of the greatest honours that I have ever had. He said that this wonderful occasion was being organised, and asked me if I would like to say something after dinner. I thought I could detect a slight note of embarrassment in his voice when he asked me if I would like to give a short scientific talk on a topic to do with hypertension. That came as a bit of a shock, and those of you who heard my talk this afternoon will no doubt have suffered a similar experience. But it is this glorious opportunity to talk about Stan, and talk with Stan and Peggy, that was irresistible. And here we all are, and I cannot imagine a nicer occasion. It is the coming together of the family, because so many of us here have spent so many years in the Medical Unit at Mary's, and we love both Stan and Peggy, so much that it really is a heart-warming time for us all. But I do not want to dwell on that too much because otherwise I shall start to be maudlin, and that is not St. Mary's style.

It is not going to be easy to get through this talk because there are some well-known hecklers about. Lever is around somewhere, and Peter Williams, is also a fair heckler, and it can be very difficult to say anything serious in the presence of some Mary's people. However, I am going to persist and start off with something serious. Then I am going to lighten it, and after that, finish up.

First I am going to talk about how I perceive Stan's scientific philosophy. He might deny it, but I think that he does actually have a scientific philosophy. Then I am going to speak about Stan's attitude to alcohol, and thirdly I shall speak about the Establishment's attitude to Stan.

First let me acknowledge a chap called Bertrand Russell. A minor English philosopher-come-mathematician-come ex-Cambridge don. Russell proposed Ten Commandments, and they are in fact the Ten Commandments of Stanley's scientific philosophy. (You must remember that I have learned these Commandments by long years of association. I am not a 'fly-by-night' associate. Stan was my Clinical Tutor in about 1954, and I did not completely leave the Medical Unit until 1972).

## The "Ten Commandments"

### No. 1:

*"Do not feel absolutely certain of anything"*

Although in a public situation when confronted, Stan seems absolutely certain, when you get close to the man he would say, "Well actually, I don't feel absolutely certain about anything".

**No. 2:**

*"Do not think it worthwhile to proceed by concealing evidence, for the evidence is sure to come to light"*

Remeber that the truth will out.

**No. 3:**

*"Never try to discourage thinking for you are sure to succeed"*

This is very important if you happen to teach at St. Mary's, and actually it is important wherever you teach.

**No. 4:**

*"When you meet with opposition endeavour to overcome it by arguement and not by authority, for a victory dependent upon authority is unreal and illusory"*

This did not always happen in the Medical Unit, although in his heart I think Stan would have liked it so.

**No. 5:**

*"Have no respect for the authorities of others, for there are always contrary authorities to be found"*

This certainly applies to Stan, and I commend it to you all.

**No. 6:**

*"Do not use power to suppress opinions you think pernicious, for if you do the opinions will suppress you"*

**No. 7:**

*"Do not fear to be eccentric in opinion, for every opinion now accepted was once eccentric"*

This certainly applies, and I think all of you who know Stan well will appreciate it.

**Nr. 8:**

*"Find more pleasure in intelligent dissent than in passive agreement, for if you value intelligence as you should, the former implies a deeper agreement than the latter"*

Being on the sharp end of a dispute with Stan is quite an experience because Stan obeys Russell's Commandment No. 8.

**No. 9:**

*"Be scrupulously truthful, even if the truth is inconvenient, for it is more inconvenient when you try to conceal it"*

("Yes, Williams, be patient, you know how many Commandments there are, for heaven's sake.")

**No. 10:**

*"Do not feel envious of the happiness of those who live in a fool's paradise, for only a fool would think it happiness"*

This final Commandment could have been spontaneously spoken by Stan.

Now that is the serious part over. Twenty years ago, Kate and I had the rewarding experience of going to Vanderbilt University in Nashville, USA, on an MRC Travelling Research Fellowship. While I was there I had a sort of desultory correspondence with Stan at various times, and in fact I had a letter back from him on one occasion, to say "Come back, all is forgotten, and there is a post in something called Clinical Pharmacology". He also kept me in touch with the domesticity of what was going on with him, and the Household, and I have this letter here, and I shall quote from it.

"The other week I had a patient who came in and presented me with a case of whisky and I took it home because whisky is whisky, and no sooner had I got to the door, than Peggy told me that she wouldn't have it in the house as it was, and I was to empty each and every bottle down the sink, or else. So reluctantly I proceeded with the unhappy task. I drew the cork from the first bottle, and poured the contents down the sink with the exception of one glass, which I drank. I pulled the cork from the second bottle and I did likewise with the exception of one glass which I drank. I emptied the third bottle, except for a glass, which I drank, and then I pulled the cork from the fourth sink, poured the glass down the bottle and drank it too. I poured the bottle from the next glass, drank one sink out of it, and I emptied the rest down the cork. Then I pulled from the next bottle, and poured it down the glass, and drank the cork, and finally I took the glass from the last bottle, emptied the cork, and poured the sink down the rest, and drank the cork. When I had everything emptied, I steadied the house with one hand, counted the bottles and glasses and

corks with the other, and found that there were 29. To make sure, I re-counted them when they came by again, this time there were 74. As the house came round the next time, I counted them again, and finally I had all the houses, and the sinks and the glasses and the corks and bottles counted, excluding one house, which I then drank. Kind regards,
Yours, Stanley."

So there you see is Stanley's attitude to alcohol. He poured it all away, which was terribly good for him.

And now, to the way that the Establishment views Stanley, and of course now we must speak of Sir Stanley and Lady Peart, and we must be properly cognisant of that honour. I entitle the following "*Ode to Stanley*" (with apologies to Stanley Holloway and Albert and the Zoo)

"T" was 7 a.m. one morning in a place called 10 Downing Street,
A lady named Margaret Thatcher was sitting bathing her feet,
On her desk was a large pile of papers
New Year's Honours for her to peruse
When she chanced upon our friend Stanley
And she called for additional views.
"I like what I hear," said Maggie
"A man of considerable worth.
One thing though you have not told me
Is concerning his Scientific research?"
She called her Scientific advisers
But they were all D.N. and A
Knowing nothing of relevant Clinical Science
So they drained to the U.S. of A.

Hidden quietly in some Glasgow tenement
An MRC Unit levered away
On Angio Aldo and Renin
It doesn't clot milk by the way.
The 'phone rang, t'was Maggie, a voice answered "Yes",
Even Margaret was somewhat put off,
But she persisted in asking her questions
That's the stuff PM's are made of.

The Sassenach was terribly helpful
Pulled out of a hat the cat's spleen
and how our Stan showed that the nerves that went into it,
Secreted nor epinephrine (noradrenaline).
"That's all very well", said Maggie,
"but what earthly use can that be.
For as things are now, with enough food and good living
we can all live till we're nigh ninety three".

An Angel appeared before her, sporting a brilliant bow tie
With the structure of angiotension tattooed upon its right thigh
"I'm the spirit of Angiotension and *actually*, I wouldn't be here
If it weren't for our young Stanley working up at Mill Hill for a year."

Now when Margaret heard that Stan worked up at Mill
She was very considerably impressed
'Cos not many people came out of t'Mill and fewer get themselves F.R. and S'ed.

The Angel went on to mention the trial on mild hypertension waxed lyrical on Stan's
early efforts with renal transplantation
If all that weren't enough the angel continued
"There are things more important than this
There's the teaching of Medicine to young and old and his style of Professorship.
There's the Wellcome, the Beit, and the Stouffer
"The Stouffer", cried Maggie, "What's that?"
Its a prize for research in America, Stan got it some years back.

"Good Lord", said Maggie, "he must work hard, nearly as hard as me"
"He does", said the Angel, "at times you know there's only him and thee".
Him and thee, in the whole of Europa, thee busy on problems of State
And him pondering the secrets of nature, like how to cure Maggie's footache.
The Angel with halo shining, went upwards terribly quick
Maggie 'phoned St. Mary's and was answered by, guess who, Gill Dick.
Gill with politest of manners, stonewalled her esteemed P.M.
For Stanley was where she knew not, without diary, or watch or pen.

But Maggie had already decided to make our Stanley a Knight
And our Peggy, already a lady, a Lady to keep him polite.
So now he's Knight and Peggy's a lady, and he's about to retire from his Chair
What will he do we wonder? Perhaps he will comb his hair?

Oh Dear, though we shall miss him, much more than we can say
No doubt that feeling of missing will wear off day by day.
Make do mistake an era is ending
Lewis, Pickering and Peart was the trend.

Now medical research is changing from mechanisms to molecular ends.
We all thought we'd be in on the final solution, but it weren't about that at all,
We were just paving the way for our friend DNA, answering a false clarion call.

So our good wishes to Peggy and the best of luck Stan
And thanks just for the chance to be here
For we've all been enriched by knowing you
And we hold you both terribly dear.
The tears that you see are real tears
They are not ashamed to be seen
Our affection will always continue
Your retirement is unreal, like a dream.
One problem I've had here in Italy
Is to find a neat rhyme for Peart
I had one nearly on my tongue
But it slipped out and was struck by a Fiat."

Ladies and Gentlemen, it is now my great pleasure to present Stanley and Peggy with
our Very Best Wishes and some gifts from us all.

Stanley, there is a card here to both you and Peggy, with signatures of almost everybody here this evening, and a commemorative programme with signatures on it.

Peggy, here is a gift for you. You are included in all our congratulations this evening, just as much as Stanley.

Stan, here is another gift for you, with our tremendous affection, and appreciation of all that you have done in many different ways for all of us here this evening.

Ladies and Gentlemen, finally, can I ask you to stand and drink a toast to Stan and Peggy.

(And a voice was heard crying "Mary's for the Cup"!)

# After dinner speech

Sir Stanley Peart

Somebody earlier today said that it would be a difficult act to follow, and I think David has proved that is likely to be true. I think I ought to tell you a few things about David, but the first thing before I set out on that task is to say how delighted we are, Peggy and I, to see you all here; you are here not only because we are retiring, but here for a very special reason, all of you; because in various ways you have touched both our lives and you have had a considerable influence on us, and I like to think in a smaller way, we have had a certain effect on you. The great pleasure for me personally has been to see that people I've thought had worth – you must agree with this! – have, in fact, justified that sort of faith, because as I look around, you are here because there is a sense of real friendliness about you all – you are not just here because you have been on the Unit or because we had a friendly relation here or there – you are here just because you have had a very special place in all our thoughts. And when I come down to the things which I value most, I feel very comforted by the fact that, as I look around, I see people who have gone on doing things on their own account and have made their own mark in medicine and science, and that is the very best thing that I have ever done by a long, long way.

Now, in terms of the serious part of the business – because you notice that we are here in Italy because both Peggy and I find Italy is – shall we say – our country. We enjoy Italy enormously, and you will notice that we have had on the Unit over the years probably more Italian research workers than most others, leaving out the Australians. The Australians have caused me more trouble than the Italians; not always very rewarding trouble either, but nevertheless they have, and I think that when you look at the record of the Italian research workers, I am absolutely delighted by the number of professors that we have had through from Italy. Over the years, it has been more difficult in the Italian academic scene for people to make their way and cling to what they thought was important to do in research. And, Alberto, if I may just reminisce a little about the first time we met. I always remember this time because it was with Cesare Bartorelli with whom Alberto used to work in Sienna. I remember we went on holiday with the children and I was dressed in shorts and a sailor shirt, I thought no matter, I will call in at St. Mary's Hospital in Sienna, because it so happens that the Sancte Maria in Sienna is named after our church and hospital in Paddington (a little matter of about 600 years between is of no consequence). So I went in, and inquired for Cesare Bartorelli and Alberto Zanchetti. After a little while they were found and immediately, to my horror, I was taken down into the bowels of the earth to find Cesare Bartorelli and Alberto Zanchetti working away, in their laboratories, in complete darkness of course. And then they said, "Well, you would like to do a ward round, wouldn't you?" I looked at myself and thought, not really, but I found myself in the unlikely position of wearing shorts and a sailor shirt trying to impress a noncomprehending Italian patient that I was some sort of an authority out of Britain; well, he could see that I obviously wasn't. But I had gained an affection for Italy then, which has never left me. I return to it with Peggy every year and one of my regrets will be missing the steady procession of Italian research workers that have come to Mary's. So when Peter and Chris, who know our love for Italy, decided this would be a good place to come, it could not have been better for us. So to Chris and Peter, who have done so much work to make this evening what it is, thank you both very much indeed.

One of the phrases I liked used by Holley Smith, who was the dean in San Francisco when I visited there some years ago, was "Behind every successful man there sits the completely astonished wife." As you know, Peggy has worn that expression in Zanchetti's photograph only too frequently. She has tried to restrain me from going over the limit of what is socially acceptable and failed!

I would like to say that there is one person I know who has worked tremendously hard on this meeting, and I know you all know it too, and that is Gerry, (Geraldine to her close friends). She has been at Mary's now for 10 years; she has put up with Peter for a shorter time than that, but nevertheless, as a working partnership they're great. And Chris, whom I first met as a Rhodes scholar at Oxford and when I saw the things he was working on, I was determined that he should come and work at some time at Mary's. And he has gone on and done great things which is another source of pleasure to me.

I have been pursued by so many wives in my time on the Unit that I just have to point out that one of the things that you have to get used to, for any of those who have aspirations to run a unit, that you do not just deal with the people working on the unit, you deal with their spouses in various ways. You get used to being rung up at three in the morning, with "Have you seen . . .? Have you heard where . . ?" and the result is no matter that you deny knowledge of where they are, you're never believed; but I got used to that.

Now finally, because you must be getting tired of the sound of my voice; I am getting tired of it myself (much to your surprise), at this table sit Paul and Renate Cottier, who are here just as Alberto is because we were in the beginning of what was then called the "Hypertension Club," which consisted of about 50 people and which first met a rather long time ago. I have a photograph of those meetings, and there was the young Paul and the young Cesare, and the young Zanchetti ("very young"). But you can reflect that that was the start of a real interest in the world in hypertension, represented just by 50 people, and now, on the whole, you could not get an international meeting under about 3000 people with an overriding interest in hypertension.

Finally, I would just like to thank Boehringer Ingelheim and their representatives here that I have known and met over many years, for their very kind support of this meeting. As you can see, it has given us all very great pleasure and between all those various relationships between the medical profession, medical research and the pharmaceutical industry I think at the bottom of it all there is a wish to help one another which is really properly based in most circumstances and I am particularly grateful this evening for that support; we all thank you for this evening.

I would just like to say once more that there is nothing that I will ever forget about this evening, the warmth that you have given both to Peggy and me by being here; taking the trouble to be here is something we will never forget and we will certainly never forget the effort that has been put into getting us all together here and may I wish you all very well in your future careers which I believe are well set on the right course, because you have got the right spirit, you have practically all got a sense of humour, you have all got a high capacity for really hard work, which is a very important entering characteristic as far as I am concerned, and you have got an international flavour which I particularly like. I feel that even if the advice I gave you was not always of the soundest, it may have acted as a cutting edge and when you were testing it drove you on to prove me wrong anyway and you got on with your careers and you have achieved so much, which is really equally as important to me as anything I have ever done myself. People like you, who are prepared, to come and wave us goodbye, or shall we say 'au revoir', have all meant a great deal in our lives and you will continue so to do. So may I just say to all of you: Thank you very much indeed.